# Domestic Violence

## How to Get Out of an Abusive Relationship

*(A Comprehensive Guide That Can Help Keep You Safer Whether You Stay or Leave)*

**Jeff Lenard**

Published By **Elena Holly**

# Jeff Lenard

*Domestic Violence: How to Get Out of an Abusive Relationship (A Comprehensive Guide That Can Help Keep You Safer Whether You Stay or Leave)*

**ISBN 978-1-998901-78-4**

Legal & Disclaimer

**Table of Contents**

## Chapter 1: My Intentions

1. To assist ladies, men and kids smash free of home violence and abuse.

Domestic violence is relegated to the shame closet - an area wherein all our darkness is sent because of guilt and societal expectancies. In order to heal, we need to remove disgrace and guilt from abuse and set ourselves and special sufferers freed from the stigma that abuse is our/their fault. It isn't your fault. Do no longer be ashamed. Do not feel accountable. Heal.

2. To offer records & help: the first-class advice constantly comes from human beings who've lived the revel in

three. To create a non-judgemental, secure area for sharing and recovery

4. To show you techniques you are in whole manage and may trade the instances of your lifestyles

five. To come up with desire and the knowledge which you are not on my own and manual is everywhere

6. To educate you a manner to allow skip of the idea that you are a sufferer. You are not a sufferer, you are not described by the usage of this, this is in fact a part of the significantly complicated person which you are

7. To show you which you need to now not popularity on the abuser (or seeking to trade/ heal them) but as an alternative on recovery your self

God, deliver me the serenity to truely take transport of the matters I can't trade, the braveness to alternate the subjects I can, and the knowledge to recognize the distinction.

- Serenity Prayer

Fortunately for me, this prayer held on our refrigerator once I modified into developing up. My step-father, the person who saved my life, have come to be a recovered alcoholic who spent some years in AA, both for remedy and as a mentor. He lived an amazing life. He achieved terrific fulfillment and then out of vicinity all of it because of his dependancy. But he regained his sobriety, worked hard and built his lifestyles lower decrease back turning into a a success entrepreneur in his very personal proper. He have become unwaveringly sincere, traumatic, right and a actual believer in me. He noticed what others did now not and understanding him modified the path of my life.

Remember, the brilliant issue you could honestly change is yourself. Be brave, love your self and realize you deserve a healthful lifestyles.

You aren't by myself. Always are searching out help. And recognise that you are endless. Anything is feasible.

"I am dwelling in hell from in some unspecified time in the future to the subsequent. But there isn't some thing I can do to interrupt out. I do not recognize wherein I may flow into if I did. I feel completely powerless, and that feeling is my jail. I entered of my very non-public free will, I locked the door, and I threw away the important thing."

- Haruki Murakami

Domestic violence and abuse isn't always your fault. You do not deserve it. No one does. But simplest YOU have the electricity to trade it. And you want to take obligation for recovery and empowering your self.

Accepting the reality that you unknowingly placed yourself within the scenario will prevent some years of unnecessary blame and victimisation.

The faster you acknowledge that you are a co-creator with the universe and that this occurred to you to reveal you genuinely how off-direction you have turn out to be, the earlier you'll heal. This acknowledgement will assist you thrive loads faster than wallowing in disgrace, guilt, blame and depression. But it's far adequate to wallow as properly - we've got were given all been there. Just do not live too lengthy.

You are powerful, never doubt that, and you have the capacity to exchange your existence and that exchange starts NOW.

Disclaimer: I am not a scientific doctor, certified counselor/therapist or psychologist. Please are seeking for assist from the suitable medical professionals for extreme and/or lifestyles-threatening issues and further useful resource.

I am teaching you a manner to heal your self based totally mostly on my personal non-public revel in. This records is supposed to empower you to take your recovery and health into your private palms. Please discover the right healthcare experts that will help you with this machine in case you revel in you want further manual.

If you are searching for assist from medical examiners, please recall consulting with domestic violence and trauma-knowledgeable professionals. Two remedies which can be examined to help trauma are: EMDR (Eye Movement Desensitization and Reprocessing) and Somatic Experiencing. Hypnosis can be powerful with the right therapist.

## Chapter 2: My Story

By the time I hit immoderate university, I turn out to be melting down. I struggled with an eating illness – bulimia – and began out to fall into the familiar entice of drinking, drugs and setting out with the wrong crowd. My correct grades disappeared, I skipped college and the bulimia have become so terrible that my mom in the long run took me to a psychiatrist.

But regardless of my psychiatrist, domestic violence and abuse have grow to be in no way noted or defined. He absolutely located me on Prozac and stated I had a chemical imbalance in my mind. He didn't understand that I changed into being physical and emotionally abused. He by no means described to me how risky and perilous my homelife absolutely have become regardless of what I told him.

Police and courts did little to intrude. After four years of court docket docket battles my parents in the long run divorced and subjects settled down. I went right now to graduate from university with honours and begin a a success career in advertising. Even in my twenties I abused alcohol to address and numb the past.

While I knew my formative years emerge as bad, I nevertheless unconsciously concept it changed into all my fault. Children don't recognize why their dad and mom damage them. They suppose there may be a few issue wrong with them. I never obtained an emotional training - I did not recognize what love felt like and I did not understand what abuse grow to be. Because of the connection with my dad and mom, I did wha such quite a few children do: confuse love with abuse.

My dad and mom in no way confirmed me love and affection, they in no way said they have been happy with me or advocated me to be glad and wholesome – but as an opportunity emotionally and physical abused me. I had no concept the way to feature healthily. I had no conceitedness and I idea I became surely damaged. Deep down, I fundamentally believed I did not deserve love and that I end up not proper enough. I had never been proven it. And I didn't have the equipment to assist myself due to the fact I turned into now not conscious that this became weird.

Finally, as quickly as I have grow to be 17 I stopped speaking to my father. I in the end were given the braveness to give up the relationship becuase I knew intuitively it did no longer serve me to spend time with him and that there has been part of him that favored to homicide my mom, brother and I. He became extraordinarily unstable and damaged.

It wasn't till I changed into in my mid-twenties that I determined what person troubles had been and the manner they contributed to abuse. After searching an investigative show about serial killer Ted Bundy, I realised that my father shared plenty of his same developments – intense narcissism (NPD) and psychopathy (Antisocial). I researched the disorder and despite the fact that this allowed me to cognitively understand that my youth abuse modified into not my fault, it did not trade subjects on my subconscious stage.

Flash beforehand to age 28, I had moved to Australia, married and given beginning to a little one boy.

Because I had no longer properly healed my abuse from early life, I had unconsciously married someone just like my dad and mom – narcissistic, showing symptoms of psychopathy and emotionally abusive.

It wasn't till after the start of my 2d infant that I knew for wonderful some thing became highly incorrect. I began out seeing psychologists, one due to the fact I suspected postnatal depression, every extraordinary to help with tension, then any other for the relationship.

All up, I visited over seven psychologists in the course of my seven-12 months marriage – even one a -hour power away – and none of them understood that I become being abused. None of them even muttered the word. Only considered one in every of them even made the relationship among my childhood and the identical styles displaying up in my marriage. I assume it had lots to do with how excessive-functioning I become – I appeared healthful, had lovely children, a wonderful profession, residence, so I didn't in shape the perceived description of domestic violence. I wasn't being crushed, but I turn out to be being abused emotionally, physical, sexually and financially.

It wasn't till my very own marriage broke down that the phrase abuse modified into ultimately located at the desk.

I turned into lower back within the US traveling own family. My husband had began an affair with a few one-of-a-kind lady, so I actually have come to be in search of to determine out what to do. I end up scared and I didn't need to move see each other psychologist, so I went to see a clairvoyant medium. She end up the primary individual who had ever stated to me, 'You are being abused and you've got got been abused your whole lifestyles.'

As fast as I heard the phrase abuse it changed into a revelation. No one had ever defined it to me. What end up abuse? What did it mean?

I came again to Australia to begin divorce court docket docket instances information that I had a elaborate conflict on my arms. I was scared for my lifestyles and the lives of my children.

No one honestly is familiar with abuse until they have got been via it. And till you name the conduct as "abuse" people often can't perceive what is and isn't always abuse. Abuse is so prevalant in our society it normalizes certainly risky behavior.

When it entails domestic violence, patients need protection and what I positioned is that police and courts aren't equipped to deal with it nicely. There were a few super establishments who helped me with DV manual whilst I even have grow to be managing safety (restraining) orders and custody, but I however felt by myself, ashamed and terrified.

What I positioned maximum distressful have become how little beneficial resource become available after the courtroom docket orders had been ultimately signed. Victims of home violence and abuse experience PTSD, or publish-traumatic stress illness, much like squaddies coming back from battle.

But in assessment to infantrymen, our war can final for many years and leave us in a consistent nation of fight-or-flight, our fitness impacted by using adrenal fatigue and burnout, and emotionally distressed while our kids maintain to visit the abusive former accomplice. A better classification is CPTSD, complex put up–worrying pressure disorder. This is closely associated with submit–annoying stress disorder, but takes region whilst a person is uncovered to extended or repeated trauma over a duration of months or years.

I become exhausted, by myself, traumatised and scared. And I knew I needed to heal, now not best from my cutting-edge divorce, however my youth. I knew that my early life come to be developing patterns in my existence that saved repeating themselves and I didn't want to stay like that anymore.

I determined to take a completely unique course and started out to paintings with healers and experts who helped me proper away heal my abuse – with the useful aid of having access to my subconscious beliefs and processing saved trauma in my frame.

These beliefs created in some unspecified time in the destiny of childhood (from the a long time of zero – 14), had laid the idea for what I might also enjoy in my grownup life. Because my adolescence emerge as abusive, I would possibly therefore experience or perpetuate abuse in some time in my life. The only way to heal it become to re-software myself and sincerely re-write my narrative and way the trauma saved in my frame.

Inspired to help others, I wrote this ebook for humans like me – who've professional abuse as a baby or in recent times left an abusive dating – and want to heal.

But I've advanced a faster manner to approach the technique. I don't need humans to spend years in speak treatment working on these things – I need you to heal speedy so that you can circulate right away to stay a outstanding lifestyles.

It's time we stopped normalising abuse and assuming that most effective positive varieties of human beings be afflicted with the aid of domestic violence – and that abuse is best bodily. Abuse takes many office work inclusive of emotional, economic, spiritual, sexual. I need to offer human beings equipment to heal themselves and empower human beings to stay their notable lives free of abuse. No one must feel ashamed or responsible approximately being abused. I want to expose them a manner to heal as fast as possible.

We moreover want to apprehend that home violence isn't always a stand-by myself hassle. Domestic violence is a symptom of an abusive society. Trying to recuperation domestic violence within the confines of a society based on abuse (energy and control over people) will not paintings. We need to restore the inspiration purpose and that might require a whole overhaul of life as we're aware about it. Imagine a society wherein truely every person are empowered, equal and violence has been eliminated because of the reality each person has the entirety they want to live on. That could genuinely remedy so plenty of our issues, together with violence in the direction of men, girls and kids.

When human beings consider domestic violence, they image a fantastic socio-monetary situation. They reflect onconsideration on people residing in poverty abusing capsules and alcohol and giving every precise black eyes. And due to their state of affairs in existence, humans assume that's truely what happens – it's a stereotype. But that isn't the handiest scenario for home violence. Domestic violence influences absolutely everyone – especially future generations. And no one deserves it, irrespective of what their state of affairs in lifestyles. And everyone want to art work together to alternate and heal it.

## Chapter 3: What Is Abuse?

According to Fleet Maull Radical Responsibility method: "... Extensively embracing one hundred% responsibility and possession of every and every circumstance you face, day in and day enjoy in your existence. This in reality goes past blame. Radical Responsibility is a trans-blame model, it's miles stepping out of the blame and disgrace paradigm all together."

"If you have got a take a look at the situations you face for your existence you may frequently see which you did have a few position in growing, allowing, or setting yourself up for these situations in a unmarried way or every other. With that perception and facts, you could then make particular alternatives which is probably going to reason specific results. By information your detail in growing a given state of affairs, you can start to choose out a way to create your future, and absolutely take possession of that."

THE NUMBERS

In america, as many as one in 4 women and one in nine men are sufferers of home violence.

In Australia, one female each week is murdered through her cutting-edge or former companion and 1 in 3 ladies and 1 in five guys have skilled at the least one incident of violence from a cutting-edge-day or former accomplice for the cause that age of 15.

Global estimates published with the aid of manner of manner of WHO mean that approximately 1 in three (35%) of girls international have expert both physical and/or sexual intimate associate violence or non-partner sexual violence of their lifetime.

Most of this violence is intimate accomplice violence. Worldwide, almost one 1/three (30%) of ladies who have been in a courting record that they've professional a few form of physical and/or sexual violence through their intimate accomplice in their lifetime.

Click under to take a look at a TED Talk with the useful resource of the use of home violence survivor and propose, Leslie Morgan Steiner.

WHAT IS DOMESTIC VIOLENCE?

Domestic violence refers to violence, abuse and intimidation among parents which can be presently or have previously been in an intimate relationship.

The wrongdoer uses violence to control and dominate the other character. This reasons worry, bodily harm and/or mental damage.

Domestic violence is a contravention of human rights.

Domestic violence consists of:

- physical attack

- sexual assault

- verbal abuse

- emotional abuse

- financial abuse

- technology-facilitated abuse

- social abuse

- non secular abuse

For me, abuse is all approximately energy and manage over others.

Abuse is described as any movement that deliberately harms or injures each extraordinary man or woman.

If we re-body abuse as energy and manipulate over others, this also shows us how abusive society and its institutions can be over us all.

Domestic violence is a symptom of a larger hassle. Abuse takes location at paintings, in schools, in hospitals and in non secular institutions, just to name a few. Abuse isn't always limited to home violence. Abuse is everywhere. We have been programmed to just accept it.

Abusers are looking for to have absolute strength and control over their patients. They save you you from residing your personal life and entrap you interior a international dominated via them. The techniques they entrap range, however generally it includes threats in competition to you and your children, inconsistent behaviour (occasionally brilliant, from time to time merciless), ensures to trade and thru the use of gaslighting (tricking you into believing you're the crazy one).

This everyday rollercoaster leaves you feeling like you are honestly trapped and there is no manner to break out them. You doubt your self. You don't apprehend what's wrong with you (as you recollect you're causing this). You assume you are the problem, no longer them. You haven't any idea what is surely taking area. It's like being out of place in a fog without a way out. And on occasion, even if you do tell a person else, they do no longer take transport of as actual with you. People who've no longer professional abuse might not recognize it.

The maximum volatile time for a girl is on the equal time as she in the long run makes a selection she does now not deserve this anymore and leaves.

ENTRAPMENT

You are trapped in an active jail or worse, possibly a literal one. You can not see a manner out and are frequently scared for your existence and the lives of your youngsters.

In some techniques, we are regularly addicted to the abuser internal the feel that we understand he/she has the potential to be splendid, so if we genuinely hold on lengthy sufficient and do everything we're capable of to make ourselves exactly what they need then possibly they'll love us and be kind to us. This will in no manner show up.

What the abuse maximum possibly represents is your dating with number one carers. As children, we had been installed upon our dad and mom to live to tell the tale. We couldn't depart them. As adults, we accept as true with the identical about our partners besides we CAN depart them. We CAN set ourselves unfastened and there may be assist available to assist us do it.

By getting rid of a person's loose will, autonomy and authenticity, abusers revel in effective. By doing so, further they entrap us.

What human beings who've professional abuse have to bear in mind is that this: abuse is handiest feasible if one individual is disempowered. If you are disempowered, you've got were given low shallowness, low self-worth and do no longer rate your self.

Of route this does not apply to each situation specifically with inclined sufferers (little one abuse, rape, random acts of violence), but in relationship abuse that is generally the case. To get away abuse you need to become empowered, rate your self and refuse to be treated badly. This takes courage and believing which you are perfect enough and you deserve the top notch for your self and/or your youngsters.

This statistics is all it takes to set you unfastened. And once this it is essential to place a plan in vicinity to make certain you and/or your youngsters are constant.

WHAT DOES ABUSE FEEL LIKE?

I'm fine it's miles excellent for every body, but abuse to me felt like dying. I felt like I became going to die at any second.

My body have become unwell and aching. I could not sleep, I couldn't devour, all I must do became worry and try to decide a manner out. I turn out to be in a consistent u . S . Of combat-and-flight. My adrenaline have come to be typically pumping. My body have come to be so tight and after I suggested humans what modified into occurring, the manner they looked at me made me revel in insane.

I modified into more scared than I had ever been in my life. I idea I will be killed - murdered - and my youngsters might be hurt, taken from me and brainwashed and abused with the useful useful resource of my abuser.

Because I changed into now not being overwhelmed, police couldn't help me - until my abuser attacked me in public and then the whole thing modified. I had witnesses. I became believed. However nonetheless no character understood except that they had skilled it.

There became assist. There were folks who ought to help me. I ultimately had been given away. But even years after the divorce and the custody papers have been signed, I modified into nonetheless scared for my life and the lives of my youngsters until I subsequently healed.

## Chapter 4: Gaslighting

Gaslighting is a form of psychological manipulation wherein a person or a fixed covertly sows seeds of doubt in a focused person, making them query their private reminiscence, perception, or judgement, often evoking in them cognitive dissonance and unique changes collectively with low self-esteem.

Using denial, misdirection, contradiction, and falsity, gaslighting involves attempts to destabilize the victim and delegitimize the sufferer's beliefs making the victim doubt themselves and their instinct. Instances may additionally variety from the denial through manner of an abuser that previous abusive incidents ever took place to the staging of peculiar activities thru the abuser with the motive of disorientating the victim

Gaslighting is so tough to understand. You love and recollect your abuser, why would they deceive you and manage you? But they do. And whilst you begin to doubt their lies and query their memories, they spin greater memories and blame you. It is the most difficult issue that can show as much as a sufferer and it takes loads time and energy to treatment all of it.

We get away abuse even as we start treating ourselves with apprehend, love and appreciation - when we honestly charge ourselves. As internal, so with out. Who we're at the inner is pondered on the out of doors. And at the same time as we change who we're at the internal, our outer truth adjustments too.

## Chapter 5: A Step-By-Step Guide For Leaving An Abusive Relationship

These are a few of the steps you may get out of an abusive dating, but continuously do what's proper for you and please stay safe

1. Find aid, get readability and ONLY surround yourself with people who trust you and recognize you're doing the right trouble.

The most essential difficulty you can do when you recognize you're being abused and in a relationship with a unstable/toxic character is to inform other human beings.

Abusers choose to abuse once they have you ever all to themselves. You need a manual organization of friends, own family and professional counselors and therapists who understand trauma and abuse.

You aren't responsible for the abuse you are experiencing—and none of the damage you're suffering is your fault. It's common for abusers to attempt to steer you that the abuse is your fault—do now not take delivery of as authentic with it.

Like every extremely good guy or women, you deserve safety, recovery, and to be preferred for who you're. If you have youngsters, you and your kids deserve a domestic freed from violence, aggression, and manipulation. You are doing the right element thru even considering leaving your abusive courting.

Once you understand you are in an abusive dating, feelings of excessive dread and anxiety can regularly take over. There is help for you, you just need to locate it and bravely gain out and ask for assist. Talk to specialists and begin to provide you with a plan. You aren't by myself.

2. Prioritise your protection as you recommend and prepare.

Your safety - and the protection of your children - is your essential assignment whilst you got out for assist and plan the way to depart an abusive relationship.

Make certain the abuser does no longer come to be conscious that you're making plans to go away. The most dangerous time for women is proper after she leaves the relationship.

Be aware about possible technology surveillance and in case you can't use your non-public mobile phone and computer, visit a library or use family or pals' gadgets to locate records and sources of help.

Change the passwords on all gadgets and keep them non-public. If you fear permitting password protection would probably draw interest from your abuser, try to advantage a clean, reasonably-priced, prepaid cellphone from the shop or ask a chum to help you get one. That can be even higher due to the reality that its lifestyles might not be diagnosed on your abuser. If your abuser can pay your cellphone invoice, it is probably satisfactory to buy your very personal cellular phone and placed it to your name.

You can also keep contacts and DV safe haven data on your new cellular telephone with out detection. After you're in a regular location and away from your abuser, you can worry approximately things like finding a contemporary location to live, finding a activity, getting counseling, and re-building your lifestyles. Getting out and being solid is your #1 precedence.

three. Talk to specialists in personal.

Do no longer speak some aspect together together with your abuser. Do no longer tell them they're abusing you. Do now not tell them you are planning to depart. Do not inform them you're looking for resource. Do now not tell them you have got were given told specific humans about your state of affairs. Keep them in the dark so you will live stable.

You want to attention on you. You need to attention on what you need to get out and live secure.

Local sufferer advocates assist you to with growing a protection plan and manual you through all of the steps of this manner. Reach out to domestic violence hotlines and network shelters so you can make sure that you can make the maximum informed picks as you navigate your scenario.

Make certain you deal with DV and trauma experts as they'll understand your situation. Not absolutely everyone is ready that will help you in the methods you want help.

If you are feeling crushed and the wait times are too lengthy, you could find out such severa super and loose materials online. You've have been given this.

4. Research nearby home violence shelters and DV help for your location.

Going to a domestic violence safe haven will offer you with the opportunity to access resources you need for the motive that they frequently come organized with clinics, counseling, legal services, and extra.

Most importantly, despite the fact that, you may be in a steady area with people who apprehend your state of affairs and what you are experiencing.

Some patients must start from scratch after leaving their abusers, and that is wherein DV shelters, victim advocates, and social employees are available in to assist them in that device and assist them become self-sufficient.

You can also be eligible for temporary financial help or unique assist to pay for vocational education to help victims attain employment and assist with relocation expenses and precise brief financial aid which consist of get right of entry to to meals and living materials.

Please allow humans help you. It's adequate to invite for assist. This is the time to permit circulate of all yourself-judgement and recognition for your fitness and safety.

five. Start saving cash.

Open your private economic group account and start putting cash into it. Keep it a secret so the abuser does now not understand it exists.

The act of saving money let you immensely as you put together to break out. If viable, bear in mind revolutionary strategies to cover and shop up cash to have on you at the same time as you leave, especially if you have to go away in a rush. Consider storing a couple of bucks consistent with week in a zipper bag hidden out of doors in a secure location.

Also don't forget having a depended on pal or loved one preserve right now to the cash for you with the particular cause to offer it once more to you while you are escaping.

The more money you can provide your self and cover out of your abuser, the higher. But please do not permit this deter you from leaving. The most crucial trouble is so that it will be solid.

Saving coins might also help you experience empowered. A lot of times, abuse includes economic manipulation. Your abuser deprives you of your private rate variety. This is entrapment. Always preserve your very non-public economic organization debts and your very very personal coins glide. Never permit a person else dictate the manner you spend coins or control whether or not or now not or no longer you have were given get right of entry to to charge range.

6. Gradually accumulate your necessities.

While your precise definition of necessity is specific to you—and may range from medicinal capsules and paperwork to kid's toys and nostalgic gadgets—it is excellent to slowly and regularly acquire the ones objects when you have the risk. That way, it may now not be apparent for your abuser which you're making plans to move away.

Make a listing of your most important objects simply so, while it's time to leave, you're capable of speedy % and depart with out traumatic approximately what to hold. In case you need to depart in a rush, you can grab what you want and go. Having a listing of devices to use as a manual can help make this way a bit a lot much less complex.

If you want to acquire those gadgets and preserve them in an unknown place (to your abuser) that is moreover a excellent idea. Just getting them out of the residence and successfully with circle of relatives and friends allow you to at the equal time as you need to head away.

Also recollect placing collectively the belongings your youngsters want to feel solid and solid. This might be hard to % away, however know-how what you want to seize if you make a hasty escape, will assist you feel greater organised and on top of things.


Remember, leaving an abuser is all approximately getting electricity and manipulate again. The extra you may do to put together the higher off you may be.

But over again, in case you want to go away and you cannot convey something with you, it without a doubt is ok too. Your protection comes first.

7. Gather your personal files.

Store your non-public statistics in a bank discipline this is great for your call or another solid vicinity far from your abuser.

Personal facts consist of:

- Birth certificates, Social Security playing cards, and so on., for you and your youngsters

- Passports

- Health insurance data and distinct scientific records

- Financial information (monetary group statements, credit score card statements, domestic mortgage, and so forth)

- Housing files (mortgage, lease/hire agreement)

- Credit document (for yourself)

- Tax returns (for yourself)

- Police critiques (if you are reporting abuse to the police)

I concealed my crucial documents in a financial organization safety container that have become handiest in my call. This manner, the documents are steady from the abuser and hearth or theft.

I moreover offered a fireplace-proof steady in which I saved other files, tough drives and information that I desired available. This ensured that I had the files that I desired, but the abuser couldn't access them. This is normally great left till you're in a steady vicinity and the abuser can't enter your property.

8. Commit to leaving and make an escape plan.

If you're inside the gadget of making the selection to go away an abusive relationship, apprehend that there are property you can flip to that will help you navigate this difficult situation.

Being afraid of now not best the abuser but the destiny is regular. It's OK to attempt to paintings at the troubles that stand up one after the alternative.

The first trouble to do is make certain you recognize all the feasible exits you may use--each door, each window. Know in advance which doors lock and the way the locks artwork, and the equal is going for domestic home windows. If you are a visible learner, draw a diagram of wherein you live and certainly mark the places you're maximum probable to physical escape from.

Once you have a smooth information of wherein you can physical go away from, write down the commands to the primary vicinity you may pass once you depart. Is it a safe haven? A buddy's residence? A family member's place of job? If possible, use the internet to discover the guidelines to that vicinity and write them down so that you do no longer need your telephone or the net to get to that area inside the future. Do the equal for a few special locations as properly.

But please ensure the abuser cannot discover this facts. You need to discover a secure region to hold these plans and facts. If it's miles too unstable, do not write a few element down.

nine. Consider getting a protection/restraining order to get rid of them from the house.

Getting a restraining/protection order is a choice to don't forget with care. It's exquisite to speak about this feature with staff at a DV steady haven, DV counselor or a criminal expert to decide what works to your specific state of affairs and times.

Depending on in which you stay and records concerning your abuser, getting a restraining order may not be the maximum consistent opportunity for you. Be powerful to talk over with a expert who can walk you through your alternatives and assist you're making the first-rate feasible selection for you.

While particular guidelines concerning restraining orders range thru kingdom, the number one device consists of going to court docket docket to document a petition, filling out workplace paintings, a form compare thru a decide, further critiques with the resource of the use of different officers, and attending a paying attention to. Eligibility to apply for an order of protection is restrained to spouses (each modern-day and those you're separated or divorced from), humans associated through blood or marriage, people you have got a baby in commonplace with, and those with which you have an intimate relationship. In all times, make sure to have a file of, and produce any documents relevant to, police reviews related to your abuser.

You can are also looking for a restraining/protection order after you are as it should be out of the residence.

10. Break the cycle and pass no touch.

Do your quality to stay as some distance away as viable out of your abuser so that you can damage the cycle. Do not contact them for any reason.

Your abuser may also try to do the whole lot they in all likelihood can to get you to go back to them. Rely on the help of family, pals, and stable haven employees to hold you targeted on what is most essential: your safety.

Even even though it'd enjoy collectively with you need your abuser in your existence, you do now not. And no matter the truth that you abuser will declare that your actions harm them, please apprehend that is most effective a recreation to play in your empathy and get you again. Stay strong. Do no longer engage.

Instead, rely upon the endless resources for humans escaping abusive relationships and permit them to help you. Not great are the ones people informed to help individuals who are for your specific situation, however they've moreover elected to be inside the ones jobs for a reason: They clearly care about your fitness, protection, and well-being. They can point you in the course of therapists, religious leaders, counselors, and such quite a few other sources an awesome manner to allow you to to your unique journey to protection and peace.

This time can be the maximum tough detail you'll ever enjoy in your life, so be affected man or woman with yourself as you navigate all of this. You're sturdy, you are courageous, and you're on the course to recuperation. Applaud your self. Be positive to take full advantage of the resources that domestic violence shelters have to offer so that you can restriction your chances of going lower back in your abuser.

# Chapter 6: How To Begin Your Healing Journey

These are the number one steps:

1. Prioritise Your Health & Safety

2. Install and Instil Boundaries

three. Saying No

four. Self-Care and Self-Love

five. Invest in Yourself

6. Remove Toxic People & Heal Codependency

7. Transform Victim Mentality

HEALTH & SAFETY

You must believe and encompass the reality that you must live a beautiful and wholesome existence. You do no longer deserve abuse.

Your safety and the safety of your children is the primary interest.

When handling home violence and abuse, typically have 1/3 sports concerned. You need witnesses - this can be police, own family or buddies.

Do now not positioned your self in situations without adult witnesses. Witnesses can maintain you safe and offer evidence in courtroom docket and most abusers will behave with different people gift. They favor to abuse you in private after which distort the truth even as you claim in any other case.

People below 18 (minors) and your children cannot function witnesses

Oftentimes, sufferers of domestic violence are charged for protecting themselves in desire to the real wrongdoer for the deliver of abuse. Make exquisite you are consistent and make sure you have not any touch with the abuser. Any contact must be in writing or through contact centres when you have youngsters.

Say no, take a look at for a home violence order/restraining order and do no longer touch the other birthday celebration for any reason. Keep your place non-public and completely off limits. You want to create a steady haven for you and your youngsters.

Do now not supply the abuser your address, change your locks, trade your cellphone amount if important (or block them from contacting you through cell cellphone or textual content) and update all passwords to banking, electronic mail and exceptional programs. If you do want to collect proof for court docket docket docket, use your vintage telephone due to the fact the manner to accumulate evidence within the intervening time purchase a trendy cellphone to apply going beforehand.

Never excuse abusive conduct. If you hear yourself pronouncing things like, "He's or she's just forced. They'll lighten up and then it's going to in all likelihood be right enough." Abuse is by no means pinnacle enough irrespective of how pressured the opposite character is at any time.

Put yourself first. You need to prove to yourself and your abuser that you could no longer tolerate abusive behaviour any more.

Remember, abuse normally follows a pattern or cycle: the tension builds, there can be conflict and then there may be a peaceful (usually that is whilst the abuser apologizes and promises to in no way do it again). Do not get caught on this cycle or agree with that the abuser will stop abusing. Get out and live away.

Remember the "definition of madness"? Doing the same aspect over and looking beforehand to important consequences (the abuser will maximum in all likelihood no longer alternate).

STAYING SAFE ACTION STEPS REVIEW

A: Call the police, find out a stable region (your private home or each different secure area) and inform every person. Abusers don't need different humans to apprehend that they will be abusing you. And in case you inform other people, your abuser may moreover launch smear campaigns to harm you and now and again declare you're the abusive one. Be organized and most significantly do no longer react to their bait or further abuse. From right here, it's miles all about disentangling yourself from them in every element.

B: Once you've got were given left, stay away. Do no longer circulate lower again. They will promise the arena to get you lower once more. Do no longer be aware of them.

C: Report all threats or abusive behaviour to police, solicitors/attorneys, counsellors, friends, family and/or a few other man or woman who will will let you. You want to shape a guide base. Build a shielding wall. You will want evidence in writing or via 1/three events. Unfortunately, courts and police may not agree with you until you have have been given evidence.

ESTABLISHING BOUNDARIES

Personal barriers are the bodily, emotional and highbrow limits we set up to guard ourselves from being manipulated, used, or violated by means of way of others. They permit us to split who we are, and what we anticipate and feel, from the thoughts and feelings of others. No touch with an abusive accomplice is step one in putting in area strong barriers.

Boundaries are what does and does no longer be definitely right for you. If you have strong limitations, people will understand how to address you. You will tell them and show them.

Here are a few pointers for putting obstacles:

-        Refuse to play the victim – you need to consciousness on empowerment

-        Determine your values: how do you want human beings to address you?

- Learn to appearance after your self first

-     Learn to surely take shipping of sadness – you can not make every body satisfied, handiest yourself

- Be ordinary with your limitations – abusers will constantly take a look at them

WHAT ARE BOUNDARIES?

You maximum possibly grew up in a family that did now not display you a manner to set up obstacles. You had no concept what became or what wasn't suitable behavior. You were probably enmeshed collectively at the side of your mother and father after which have grow to be enmeshed collectively along side your companions. Where you stop and they start may be hard to determine.

Learning a way to installation barriers is the number one manner to preserve your former companion, and future companions, from taking advantage of, or hurting you. And remember, you cannot manipulate your abuser. The great man or woman you may control is yourself.

TASK: WHAT ARE SOME BOUNDARIES YOU NEED TO ENFORCE? MAKE A LIST.

Boundaries are what you train kids. Boundaries are what you train abusive adults (who're basically in fact raging kids on the indoors).

No contact with an abusive accomplice is kind of usually important and studying how not to react to their bait and reply in a comfortable, business enterprise-like way will educate them that you aren't at their mercy. If you can't be manipulated and controlled, they may in the long run give up and locate a person else to abuse.

But as quickly as you located up limitations the abuser will take a look at to look how robust they absolutely are. KEEP THEM STRONG! And stay ordinary.

SAYING NO

Learning how to mention no and rise up for yourself with out feeling disgrace or guilt is important on your healing. You need to put your self first no matter what. People will no longer love you or such as you extra in case you are a consistent giver, they will truely take increasingly more.

Many sufferers of abuse were professional as kids to emerge as humans-pleasers and doormats, therefore, we discover it tough to mention no to humans and situations that aren't in our excellent interest.

If we constantly placed particular humans first, then due to this we are putting ourselves final. This comes from our capability to empathise with each person and all and sundry. But this hyperactive empathy muscle does not serve us. We need to begin doing topics which can be in our quality interest.

DO YOU KNOW WHAT WORKS FOR YOU AND WHAT DOESN'T? MAKE A LIST.

SELF-CARE + SELF-LOVE

One of the motives we find out ourselves in relationships that harm us is due to our exposure to abuse in children.

Our subconscious programming from some time 0 – 14 determines how we stand up relationships, jobs, conditions, and the whole lot else in life besides we consciously clean the testimonies and emotions, change our beliefs and re-write the packages.

If we have an abusive person in our life which means that we may also moreover have an abusive individual internal folks (our mum and dad internalised and writing our internal script).

Not most effective are we being abused at the out of doors, but we also are abusing ourselves at the inner with essential self-talk, self-sabotage and by using using surrounding ourselves with toxic folks that do not sincerely love and assist us.

Only on the same time as we shift our internal global via self-love and self-care do we begin to see our outer worldwide shift as properly.

Find approaches to connect with your self. Take an stock of the ways you hurt yourself and begin changing your internal speak to be supportive in vicinity of important.

Start to understand the patterns from your youth that were furthermore found for your abusive dating.

Are there common topics that seem to replicate themselves in all your relationships?

Did your abuser remind you of a number one carer?

## SELF-CARE AND HEALING AFTER TRAUMA

After experiencing home violence, you also are physical and mentally stricken by PTSD (post-traumatic stress illness) and/or CPTSD (complex publish-worrying stress disorder). If you want to create a higher life, you want to discover ways to placed your self first, cope with your self, love your self, heal codependency by means of manner of becoming responsible and unbiased, and heal the trauma from the abuse you have got have been given suffered sooner or later of your lifetime.

If you want to exchange your outer reality, first we should trade our inner reality. Learning a manner to sluggish down, regulate your fearful system, calm your feelings and call your frame is a first-rate manner to start the method. Treat your self like a loving decide who cares for their toddler. It's your turn to be loved and nourished.

- Connect with friends and own family who love and help you

- Exercise - yoga, health club, health instructions

- Get massages or other kinds of recovery frame work

- Meditate - or circulate for a walk or perform a touch gardening

- Remove caffeine and alcohol from your weight loss plan and discover ways to modify your worried device

- Eat healthy food and keep away from sugar

- Laugh and have fun

INVEST IN YOURSELF

Do the subjects which you've typically favored to do - it's a brand new beginning and you subsequently have the liberty to be who you are alleged to be.

Learn new talents, empower yourself, and construct a network round you that allows your recuperation and thriving.

Find guide for your kids via counsellors and first rate characteristic models and be the great figure you'll be.

Always play the lengthy activity – make the abuser appear like the abuser they'll be via turning into your outstanding self.

By making an investment in yourself, you're telling the universe you're worthy of an incredible existence and also you ought to be treated with love and respect. The extra you invest in yourself, the better your lifestyles turns into.

What are a few skills you want to investigate? Are there commands you'd like to take? Music/plays/movies you would really like to look? Bucket listing objects you want to tick off? Now is the time to do YOU!

TOXIC PEOPLE

After leaving an abusive relationship DO NOT START DATING OR SEEING OTHER PEOPLE. You need time to properly heal, grieve and get to comprehend your self. Delete the connection apps and as an alternative date your self.

If you aren't healed, you can attraction to poisonous human beings lower back into your lifestyles and repeat the sample. Toxic people encompass strength vampires, narcissists/sociopaths/psychopaths (lack empathy, sell selfishness, violence), bad Nellies and chaos addicts – do not play their exercise.

In reality, every body who does now not uplift you and convey pinnacle topics into your existence needs to move. Friends and circle of relatives who display poisonous behaviour furthermore need to be eliminated from your lifestyles on the identical time as you heal. You need to focus all of your strength on your self and ensure you have got region to heal.

Cutting Cords: It's moreover an tremendous concept to cut energetic cords. Often, even when we physically leave an abuser, we are though energetically connected to them. By disposing of the strength cord that binds you to any other individual you could not feed power to them.

To cut cords you want to visualise your electricity challenge and ask your SPIRIT to lessen any inlays or outlays amongst you and your abuser. Physically use your hands to lessen those cords and then pull them out on the idea. Repeat as important until you experience the electricity change and lighten.

WHAT IS CODEPENDENCY?

Codependency is a trauma response from early life. Our number one caregivers educate us that a good way to be cherished we need to abandon or sacrifice our actual self. We use this statistics to form our relationships and are often inquisitive about narcissists and exclusive human beings with additions.

Co-dependents sacrifice themselves for others. They are complete-time martyrs.

The remarkable definition I've determined for codependency is from Dr. Becky Whetstone:

"Co-dependents are relationally immature to the type of degree that it hampers their existence and relationships over-and-all over again.

It want to be said which you don't should be from an brazenly abusive circle of relatives to have been traumatized — the principle requirement is which you took on disgrace at one issue that brought about you to have the crucial middle belief that, 'There is a few factor wrong with me, or I'm faulty.'

Once someone concludes that they are faulty they exchange themselves to seize up on the issues they experience that they have. Therein lies co-dependence. A man or woman turns into 'developmentally immature,' or co-based, the moment they lose themselves in youngsters and morph into a few sort of faux self, together with a pleaser, rebel, perfectionist, bully, controller, clown, or any shape of person that isn't the real, actual self."

SYMPTOMS OF CODEPENDENCY

Primary signs and symptoms of co-dependency include:

- Difficulty experiencing suitable levels of shallowness, because of this, and hassle loving the self.

- Difficulty setting functional barriers with specific human beings. You have trouble protecting the self (humans-appealing, can't say no).

- Difficulty proudly proudly owning one's personal truth accurately. You have hassle identifying who one is and understanding a manner to percent that correctly with others.

- Difficulty addressing interdependently one's individual want and desires. You have hassle with self-care.

- Difficulty experiencing and expressing one's truth carefully, (are you controlling or out-of-

manipulate?). You have problem being suitable for one's age and severa occasions.

To heal from codependency, we want to engage assist via a twelve-step utility and treat this as an dependancy. Please looking for expert assist. The intention is to area yourself first, love yourself, invest in your self and learn how to use your boundaries and say no. Codependency, in my view, is one of the essential reasons why we come to be in violent and abusive relationships.

CODEPENDENCY & ADDICTION

Codependency, like drug and alcohol abuse, is an addiction and there are twelve-step packages. I in particular recommend the ones for clearly every body who have become in an abusive dating. As patients, we are able to regularly end up "addicted" to the abuser and their abuse. This is why it is so tough for us to go away. We realize it's far horrible for us, however we flow into lower decrease back for added. We preserve to the concept that they will change and love us once more. But that is a faux wish and only an addiction.

If we aren't cherished as kids, we will have problem forming healthy, loving relationships as adults. Co-dependents are children who took on trauma and disgrace and in no manner felt cherished – or worse yet, felt as notwithstanding the fact that there has been a few thing incorrect with them which made them unloveable. Co-dependents are martyrs – we will do anything as long as we assume our accomplice might love us – or at the least no longer abandon us. And like alcoholism and drug abuse, it is an dependancy.

Think about it this manner, as kids we attempted the entirety in our energy to emerge as loveable. That didn't art work so we strive the entirety in our electricity to be loveable in our relationships. Which once more doesn't artwork. What we must do is simply love and rate ourselves and encompass the belief that we're worth.

This internal rate and worthiness will keep us out of poisonous relationships and codependency. We will ensure to vicinity ourselves first.

Besides our early youth relationships, culture is also in fee. Movies, books, song and tv indicates idealise addictive relationships. People have come to trust that their "first-rate" mate will complete them, make lifestyles well well worth dwelling, or otherwise take a meaningless lifestyles and make it extra worthwhile.

# Chapter 7: Personality Disorders & Domestic Violence

Why may additionally we fall in love with an abuser? Because of what we professional in youngsters. And a few element known as 'trauma bonding.'

We subconsciously are searching out out people who reflect what we professional in early life and this 'acquainted familial bond' keeps us trapped inner the dangerous courting. We can also moreover call it love at the beginning, but after the honeymoon period is over, abuse gadgets in.

Most frequently than now not, abusers may be categorised into the following forms of personality issues:

- Borderline Personality Disorder

- Narcissistic Personality Disorder

- Antisocial Personality Disorder (aka sociopathy/psychopathy)

- Paranoid Personality Disorder

It's a superb concept to be able to pick out what sickness your abuser possesses (every now and then multiple) so you can plan for that reason, learn how to anticipate unique behaviour and keep away from those human beings in the destiny.

The Narcissist and the Empath: A Match Made in Hell

Polarities: the Narcissist & the Empath form a trauma bond based on what they skilled as children.

One selected severe empathy and self-sacrifice (the empath) as a way to address trauma and abuse, the alternative near down empathy and compassion and determined on to sacrifice others to deal with trauma and abuse (narcissist).

Both are patients of negative adolescents environments and each conditions are similarly as damaging.

The empath will trying to find out narcissists so that it will heal his or her early life enjoy and caregivers.

The narcissist will are looking for the empath due to the truth he or she is aware of they could have energy and control over them. And deep down they crave the connection with the father or mother that they in no way had and the empath so needlessly materials.

The narcissist seeks unconditional love, adoration and guide. The empath seeks people who need their affection and self-sacrifice.

Task: List all of the approaches you sacrificed yourself for romance.

BORDERLINE PERSONALITY DISORDER

Borderline man or woman disease is a important intellectual circumstance that's characterised via unstable moods and feelings, relationships, and conduct.

Borderline character ailment signs encompass instability in interpersonal relationships, self-picture, and emotion, similarly to a sample of impulsive behaviors.

Signs and signs and symptoms and signs and symptoms and signs embody:

- Fear of abandonment

- Unstable relationships (warfare, neediness)

- Identity Impairment (low shallowness, low self esteem)

- Impulsive behaviour (spending, sex, binging, law breaking, and so on)

- Self-damage/ suicide

- Emotional instability

- Feeling of emptinessIntense anger and and aggressive behaviour

If you are in, or had been in a dating with a person who suffers from BPD, it is like using a roller coaster – you in no way apprehend what to expect.

NARCISSISTIC PERSONALITY DISORDER

Narcissistic personality disease — virtually one among numerous kinds of man or woman problems — is a mental condition wherein humans have an inflated experience in their private significance, a deep want for immoderate attention and admiration, troubled relationships, and a lack of empathy for others. But inside the again of this masks of extreme self warranty lies a delicate vanity that's susceptible to the slightest grievance.

Narcissistic character infection motives issues in many regions of life, which consist of relationships, paintings, college or financial affairs. People with narcissistic persona sickness can be commonly unhappy and disappointed once they're no longer given the precise favors or admiration they believe they deserve. They may additionally discover their relationships unfulfilling, and others won't revel in being spherical them.

Signs and symptoms and symptoms of narcissistic individual disorder and the severity of signs and symptoms and signs and symptoms range. People with the ailment can:

- Have an exaggerated feel of self-importance

- Have a experience of entitlement and require normal, immoderate admiration

- Expect to be diagnosed as superior even without achievements that warrant it

- Exaggerate achievements and talents

- Be preoccupied with fantasies approximately achievement, strength, brilliance, splendor or the first-class mate

- Believe they're superior and can handiest accomplice with further special people

- Monopolize conversations and belittle or appearance down on humans they understand as inferior

- Expect particular favors and unquestioning compliance with their expectancies

- Take advantage of others to get what they want

- Have an inability or unwillingness to recognize the desires and feelings of others

- Be inexperienced with envy of others and endure in thoughts others envy them

- Behave in an smug or haughty way, discovering as conceited, conceited and pretentious

- Insist on having the fantastic of everything — as an instance, the tremendous automobile or office

At the equal time, humans with narcissistic individual ailment have hassle dealing with some aspect they recognize as criticism, and they could:

- Become impatient or irritated when they don't get preserve of precise treatment

- Have sizable interpersonal problems and effortlessly sense slighted

- React with rage or contempt and attempt to belittle the other character to make themselves appear advanced

- Have problem regulating feelings and behavior

- Experience primary troubles dealing with stress and adapting to exchange

- Feel depressed and moody because of the fact they fall brief of perfection

- Have thriller emotions of loss of confidence, shame, vulnerability and humiliation

ANTISOCIAL PERSONALITY DISORDER

Antisocial man or woman illness, every now and then called sociopathy/psychopathy, is a mental circumstance wherein someone constantly shows no regard for right and incorrect and ignores the rights and feelings of others. People with antisocial character illness have a propensity to antagonize, manage or deal with others harshly or with callous indifference. They display no guilt or regret for their behavior.

Individuals with antisocial character ailment frequently violate the regulation, turning into criminals. They can also additionally moreover lie, behave violently or abruptly, and characteristic troubles with drug and alcohol use. Because of these traits, people with this sickness normally can't satisfy obligations related to own family, art work or college.

Antisocial individual disorder signs and symptoms and signs and symptoms might also moreover encompass:

- Disregard for proper and incorrect

- Persistent mendacity or deceit to make the most others

- Being callous, cynical and disrespectful of others

- Using enchantment or wit to govern others for personal benefit or private delight

- Arrogance, a experience of superiority and being highly opinionated

- Recurring issues with the regulation, which include crook behavior

- Repeatedly violating the rights of others through intimidation and dishonesty

- Impulsiveness or failure to plot in advance

- Hostility, high-quality irritability, agitation, aggression or violence

- Lack of empathy for others and absence of remorse approximately harming others

- Unnecessary risk-taking or volatile behavior without a regard for the safety of self or others

- Poor or abusive relationships

- Failure to bear in mind the horrible effects of conduct or observe from them

- Being usually irresponsible and repeatedly failing to meet paintings or financial responsibilities

Adults with delinquent character sickness normally display symptoms and signs of conduct ailment in advance than the age of 15. Signs and symptoms and symptoms of conduct ailment consist of severe, chronic behavior problems, which encompass:

- Aggression within the path of humans and animals

- Destruction of assets

- Deceitfulness

- Theft

- Serious violation of guidelines

PARANOID PERSONALITY DISORDER

People with PPD are commonly on guard, believing that others are constantly looking for to demean, damage, or threaten them. These normally unfounded ideals, in addition to their behavior of blame and distrust, can also additionally intrude with their capability to form near relationships.

People with this disorder:

- Doubt the willpower, loyalty, or trustworthiness of others, believing others are the use of or deceiving them

- Are reluctant to divulge heart's contents to others or show personal information because of a worry that the records can be used in the direction of them

- Are unforgiving and maintain grudges

- Are hypersensitive and take complaint poorly

- Read hidden meanings in the innocent feedback or informal seems of others

- Perceive attacks on their character that aren't apparent to others; they usually react with anger and are brief to retaliate

- Have recurrent suspicions, without reason, that their spouses or enthusiasts are being untrue

- Are usually cold and some distance off in their relationships with others, and can become controlling and jealous

- Cannot see their position in issues or conflicts and recall they'll be commonly proper

- Have hassle enjoyable

- Are damaging, stubborn, and argumentative

The actual motive of PPD is not stated, however it probably consists of a aggregate of organic and mental elements. The truth that PPD is more common in people who have near loved ones with schizophrenia suggests a genetic link between the two issues. Early early life research, which embody physical or emotional trauma, also are suspected to play a function inside the improvement of PPD.

## Chapter 8: Victim Mentality

What if I recommended you that irrespective of what, you aren't a sufferer?

That as an possibility, you are a creator of your reality.

And that everything that has came about to you or will display as a good deal as you modified into created through the use of you every consciously and unconsciously or a result of cause and effect?

"It's psychologically wholesome to widely known the suffering and feelings of powerlessness that accompany stressful studies. And however, there are those those who experience like patients all of the time, irrespective of their instances. Those with a victim mentality are constantly being victimized, as a minimum of their very very own mind. They preserve a everyday victim identity and spot life thru constantly sufferer-tinted glasses" (Psychology Today).

The definition of a sufferer is a person who has been attacked, injured, robbed, killed, cheated, or fooled through manner of someone else, or harmed with the useful resource of manner of an unpleasant event. Everyone is a victim of some aspect in a few unspecified time within the future. The aim is to now not stay one, but faucet into resilience.

Abuse is not your fault. But as a survivor you want to just accept the state of affairs, take duty for it, actively heal your self, create a assist network and cast off poisonous human beings from your lifestyles.

Continuing to be a victim and blame the abuser does now not paintings. You have to take actionable steps to unfastened yourself from the pattern of abuse.

The perpetual victim makes use of blame to deflect feeling lousy approximately oneself. By doing away with blame for their behaviour, it liberates them from having to grow to be aware of with the effects of their movements.

They blame others and the sector for his or her cutting-edge events. They do not anticipate possession in their lives considering to accomplish that could suggest managing uncomfortable feelings which threaten their vanity.

We are patients of domestic violence however now not for all time. Once we go away the abuser, and take control of our very own lives, we aren't sufferers - we should emerge as EMPOWERED.

While it's miles adequate to inform people what took place and really very own and recognize your tale, do no longer allow it outline you or use it as a manner to avoid healing and supporting yourself. To actually heal from home violence and abuse, you need to now not pick out as a victim but as a survivor.

# Chapter 9: What Is Trauma And How To Heal It

Trauma is so misunderstood.

We often mistakenly accept as true with that trauma is constantly an immoderate bodily event or damage which encompass a vehicle accident, gunshot or deceased loved one. But trauma isn't constrained to or defined thru its "period" or context.

Trauma may be as diffused as someone telling you which you "look fat" or as large as being held hostage at gunpoint. The way we enjoy, interpret and react to any and all traumas determines how a good deal they have got an impact on us.

Trauma is described as any experience – no matter how large or small – that disconnects us from our real "self." Also, any experience that dysregulates our feelings, thoughts, body, fitness or spirit is considered trauma.

Traumas software program us to use protective techniques to preserve us strong. These strategies, which might be stored in our frame and aggravating device, do maintain us safe, but they can also cross into overdrive and prevent us from experiencing and carrying out what we choice in existence.

Trauma can seem as emotions of regular states of combat-flight-freeze, anxiety, flashbacks, melancholy or looping (same styles offering on your existence time and again all over again).

DOMESTIC VIOLENCE & TRAUMA

Domestic violence in fact includes trauma - every physical and emotional trauma - that receives trapped in each the bodily and emotional bodies. Trauma is an energetic problem as well as a bodily trouble (physical it is stored in our autonomic anxious device - energetically it is stored in our power/emotional problem).

It can preserve us stuck - despite the fact that we go away the relationship - it is able to show up in our bodies through numerous sicknesses and health issues, and in order for us to heal well, we should art work on processing and clearing trauma.

Trauma places us on a repeat loop and prevents us from co-developing with the universe as we're now not capable of shipping via time and location. Not most effective does it rob us of our past, however it may furthermore steal our destiny if we leave it unhealed.

Survivors of Domestic Violence Suffer From:

Post-Traumatic Stress Disorder and Complex Trauma

Post-traumatic pressure disorder (PTSD) is a intellectual fitness situation added on thru the usage of a terrifying event — each experiencing it or witnessing it.

Symptoms also can embody flashbacks, nightmares and immoderate anxiety, further to uncontrollable thoughts about the event.

Most folks who experience worrying activities can also have brief trouble adjusting and coping, however with time and suitable self-care, they normally get better. If the symptoms worsen, last for months or possibly years, and interfere along with your daily functioning, you could have PTSD.

For survivors of domestic violence, PTSD isn't always like someone who has been in an twist of fate or at battle. We are abused by using the usage of dad and mom which is probably speculated to love us - own family, companions -

so this critically impairs our potential to really be given as genuine with ourselves in addition to special humans and might intervene with our capability to shape healthful relationships. That is why our trauma is a mix of PTSD and complicated trauma.

Complex Trauma Disorder

Complex trauma can rise up at some point of adolescence or maturity - it's miles occasionally known as Childhood PTSD. Most survivors of domestic violence actually be with the resource of complex trauma, no longer just PTSD.

It is an enjoy of repeated disturbing occasions over an extended time period consisting of abuse or neglect approximately, or social trauma which incorporates conflict or cultural dislocation. Its results on intellectual and bodily fitness may be extended-lasting – impacting on emotional health, well-being, relationships and every day functioning.

This is the trickiest trauma to cope with and the least understood. Not nice does this trauma get stored to your body, but it additionally rewires your mind and forestalls it from functioning normally. Healing this shape of trauma requires a somatic, intellectual (neuroplasticity) and lively approach.

What Happens After Trauma?

It's one-of-a-type for anyone and is based upon at the person and the severity and length of exposure to the trauma. Some humans should experience:

• emotional numbness and detachment – feeling reduce off from what occurred, unique humans, and yourself

• marvel and disbelief – that the event befell

• worry – of demise or damage, being by myself, not being capable of cope, or the occasion taking region another time

• helplessness – feeling which you have no manipulate

• avoidance – of factors that remind you of the event

• poor mind or emotions – about the area or the reaction to the occasion

• modifications in relationships – feeling faraway from others.

• guilt or disgrace – for no longer having stopped the event, or for being better off than others, or for not reacting higher or coping nicely sufficient

• unhappiness – for topics that have prolonged long gone or been misplaced

•isolation – feeling that no person is familiar with or can assist

• pride – remedy at being alive and solid

• anger and frustration – about the event, or the unfairness of it

• re-experiencing the event – through dreams, flashbacks or thoughts

What are the Long-Term Effects After PTSD and CPTSD?

The long-time period effects of post-annoying pressure illness can embody the subsequent:

• complications

• adjustments in urge for food and weight

- racing coronary heart

- shaking or sweating

- trouble sleeping

- trouble concentrating

- emotional changes, like mood swings, tension, or a short temper

- issue with college or paintings

- withdrawal from pals and circle of relatives

- problems preserving up with normal each day sports

- threat-taking, together with extended use of alcohol and different drugs

- being overly alert or watchful

- reminders of the stressful occasion which can be distressing. These can also need to encompass: desires, flashbacks, thoughts or memories of the event coming decrease back unexpectedly, physiological reactions that remind you of the event

• fending off topics that remind you of the event. This can consist of keeping off particular people, places, or activities. It also can encompass efforts to avoid any unwanted memories, mind or emotions

PTSD also can reason changes on your mood and questioning. For instance those can include vital changes to beliefs about oneself, others or the area, similarly to primary changes to your emotional country (that gets inside the manner of residing the life you need to live).

Unresolved Trauma and Stored Survival Stress

Unresolved trauma often suggests up in styles. No remember variety what we do, we maintain getting the equal give up result.

Three subjects that regularly element to unhealed trauma are:

1. Continually terrible outcomes and sabotage styles

2. Inability to deal with emotional triggers and crush

three. Unhealthy our our bodies (autoimmune ailments, pores and pores and pores and skin troubles, aches and pains, and lots of others)

4. Turbulent relationships

Because our concerned machine is so pressured with the unhealed trauma, we're continuously in combat, flight or freeze. This trauma manifests itself in our fact and through looking at our lives and what constantly shows up (patterns) this could lead us to treating and recovery our trauma.

TASKS: WHAT KEEPS SHOWING UP IN YOUR LIFE?

WHAT ARE SOME WAYS YOU KEEP SABOTAGING YOURSELF OR KEEPING YOURSELF STUCK TO STAY SAFE?

ARE YOU SUFFERING FROM ANY AUTO-IMMUNE OR HEALTH ISSUES?

For instance, allow's test your abusive ex-partner:

Why did you fall in love with this man or woman?

Did they remind you of a person?

Once you have been inside the courting after a few years, did they start to show off behaviour similar to behavior from one in every of your parents?

Do you entice human beings into your lifestyles that mirror your relationship at the side of your dad or mum?

We all experience one-of-a-kind childhoods. And whatever we experience informs the imprint of our unconscious from the ages of zero-14. From those imprints, we then co-create our fact.

To understand the imprints on your unconscious, you have to start to apprehend styles in your existence and ask the question 'in which did this come from?' Most likely it's without delay associated with an experience out of your early life a few of the a long time of zero-14.

Healing Trauma

If, like me, you skilled trauma and abuse some of the a long term of 0-14, then your unconscious is developing an experience for you that indicates that - this is why we come to be with abusive partners. It can also hyperlink decrease returned to a beyond lifestyles! I understand, crazy proper!

I met my abusive ex in numerous of my very own beyond lives.

If we need to create a healthy, satisfied existence, we want to reprogram our unconscious, smooth our past lifestyles revel in and heal - and bet what? It's clean to do!

Using Belief Hacking™ to Heal Trauma

Trauma is an electricity (emotion + enjoy = stress) that gets trapped for your body, autonomic worried tool and strength fields.

Instead of preserving homeostasis, sufferers from PTSD/CPTSD hold to experience trauma regardless of what they do. Sufferers continuously experience fight-flight-freeze -fawn (dysregulation of the sympathetic involved machine) which over an extended time frame, can harm down a wholesome body and in the end create sickness and one-of-a-kind illnesses.

Trauma may be cleared from the physical body and lively our our bodies the use of a combination of BELIEF HACKING™, mindfulness, breathwork, diet and life-style modifications.

What we do recognize is that trauma affects surely all of us otherwise and counting on the diploma and frequency of trauma its results variety.

To free this trapped electricity (trauma), there are a number of approaches to technique restoration, however I've located that none of them are as brief and effective as BELIEF HACKING™.

What is Belief Hacking™?

Based by myself non-public revel in and education, the quickest and handiest manner to heal trauma, is to use a modality I created called BELIEF HACKING™. BELIEF HACKING™ clears the experience, feelings, ideals and trauma from our bodily bodies, lively field and time-song (past, gift and destiny)

We are multidimensional beings in a multidimensional worldwide with invisible active factors, together with meridians, chakras, auras, spirits and souls, further to the bodily body and all its organs. All mind and ideals are invisible, but they are nevertheless energy. By using quantum restoration, we unfold time and smooth the trauma from their revel in at the inspiration cause.

The root motive is usually an enjoy that occured among the a while of 0-14 - however normally, traumas and opinions in our existence additionally link lower lower back to past lives. We also can clear the trauma from beyond lives which is probably affecting you currently.

BELIEF HACKING™ works with the aid of having access to the size wherein the trauma (root reason) have become first created and clearing it. BELIEF HACKING™ speedy and with out hassle gets rid of trapped energy, feelings, trauma and proscribing beliefs from the frame and unconscious mind. BELIEF HACKING™ accesses the premise cause using the frame's data tool (the unconscious) to pinpoint the primary age in this lifetime a stressful or terrible imprinting revel in occurred.

When we enjoy a trauma – that event and our response to it (emotions + beliefs) – can emerge as trapped in our body and power issue it is why we enjoy as despite the fact that we "in no way had been given over it" or the effects appear to seem to us over and over once more. This is likewise known as "looping" as it seems like (to our our bodies) that the trauma keeps occurring time and again.

Or it could be induced off with the beneficial resource of some thing or someone acquainted.

For example, as a baby you can had been "disciplined" harshly with the aid of way of way of a parent. Along with this physical abuse, you lock in the feelings of fear, anger and devastation amongst others. The ideals you lock in might be "I'm horrible" or "I'm no longer worthy of affection." These feelings and ideals can grow to be "frozen" in time and activated on every occasion you enjoy you're being "punished" for not "following the policies."

In the destiny, this measurement of time is brought on off, for this reason preserving you looping into this kingdom of fear, anger and devastation collectively with the beliefs "I'm awful" and "I'm no longer well worth of affection" similarly to the unconscious understanding that if "I don't have a study the policies and do as I'm counseled, I can be punished." We don't need that! That's why it's so important to recognize your subconscious notion machine and easy and heal your restricting beliefs.

# Chapter 10: We Are The Technology (And The Magic)

"Any sufficiently advanced era is indistinguishable from magic."

- Arthur C. Clarke

Through advent (or manifestation) we remodel energy from the ethers (non-fabric nation-states) into bodily (and every so often non-physical) gadgets in our fact. Our inner worldwide takes bodily shape. If we preferred to apprehend who we're and the manner we paintings, wouldn't it make enjoy to create it?

I'm not most effective 100% religious - I'm moreover a hundred% functional.

If we take a look at the generation we create, the solutions to how we paintings are all round us.

We're Kind of Like Computers

Despite our medical improvements, we nevertheless have no longer responded the questions: who're we and why are we right right here? And counting on what human beings take delivery of as real with, all of us have one-of-a-kind answers.

Based on the studies I've achieved and my very personal non-public journeys, what I recognize is this: we're right proper here to comply reputation thru embodiment. And to enjoy love and joy. That's it. It's smooth. It's actually laughable how very complex we make existence and what type of suffering we inflict on ourselves and others.

We are also super creators. We are given the gives of introduction, however free will permits us to select what we create.

And what we need to be aware of is how effective disembodied attention (artificial intelligence, augmented reality, digital fact, and lots of others) is and the way detrimental it is able to be. Humans have an top notch functionality for romance, compassion and empathy which all comes from our coronary coronary heart. Intelligence with out this coronary coronary heart-thoughts connection – whether it's far residing in a body or now not – is unstable. This is what makes narcissists and psychopaths so unstable - they may be disconnected from their coronary coronary heart.

But as we create this splendid new era, we need to apprehend that those enhancements are education us about how we paintings, how we're made and how our very own generation lets in us to function.

How We Work

We are most like quantum pc structures – we can be in severa locations without delay and in ourselves are our non-public universe.

We have a soul and spirit and we are strolling with pretty a few energy (the seven chakras) and our bodies: physical, lively, emotional and highbrow.

There are also our beyond lives – or parallel lives – taking place concurrently as time isn't always linear, it is taking region abruptly. But our lifetimes do run in a pretty sequential order. Many times, the issues we are having in our current-day lifestyles, link decrease returned to some issue that befell in a past lifestyles.

In every incarnation of existence (each lifetime) we have were given precise mother and father, as a end result awesome biology, for that reason a fantastic soul. Our soul is anchored in or to our our bodies and stories our lives in my opinion. We have many tremendous souls residing many unique lives thru time. Our soul is kind of a pc/computer.

Spirit links our souls to every one-of-a-kind and to God/Source (the strength that allows us to exist on this universe). Spirit is the source of all life - the entirety has a spirit (but now not the entirety has a soul).

Working with Spirit

The existence strain — the technology that connects us thru time and region further to our separate incarnations — is our Spirit (a few humans talk with this as superconscious). Spirit does not exchange with each life; it's far the only steady.

Our Spirit publications us and connects us similar to the internet. The internet connects to man or woman laptop structures and creates a community. This community connects to other computer systems and databases everywhere in the global. Our Spirit is attached to all our souls via time and region. Spirit is likewise related to supply — or the place in which everyone come from (some thing that is probably).

Spirit may additionally even help us similar to how Siri lets in us navigate our smartphone. We can ask Spirit questions and we will command Spirit to make adjustments to our power and our our bodies.

For example, once I go to bed each night time time, I ask my Spirit to easy all the power from my subject and body that I skilled that day.

Shamans have labored with and used Spirit for loads of years. This isn't a extremely-modern-day technology. Just new to us.

Viruses and Faulty Programming

Have you ever clicked on an electronic mail and by using twist of fate downloaded spyware or a pandemic? We do the equal detail with our power all the time.

Whenever we decrease our protective strength hassle through low vibration feelings (unhappiness, despair, exhaustion), sex without love, drugs and alcohol, disease and malnutrition, we open ourselves to entity invasion. Nergetic beings from unique dimensions can bounce into our energy fields and every manage us or feed off our energy. We can also allow this whilst we name in topics which incorporates gods, goddesses, aliens or special entities thru ritual. This is common some of the New Age movement.

Like a computer, we run sure applications primarily based on what we studies, enjoy, suppose and take delivery of as genuine with.

'Programs' encompass our dad and mom' belief structures, wherein we develop up (beliefs about race, socioeconomic reputation, gender), faith, college, government, way of lifestyles, and masses of others. These packages form us and mould us and stress ideals into us that aren't our private.

So many of the packages and the viruses (horrific downloads) on occasion it's far not possible to surely embody our real selves. Experiencing trauma can without a doubt motive us to crash our structures. We down load viruses and our programming receives surely scrambled. This is why it is so vital to heal our trauma, rewrite the vintage packages and bring our our our bodies and strength lower again into balance.

Optimising Ourselves

This is what I recognise for high-quality: we come to Earth lifetime after lifetime to adapt (flow into through time) and create. We are every unique and unique with super gives to percentage. Death is not the stop, it's miles only a transition. We live below the well-known law of purpose and impact (karma). If this, then that. Which way that what you do unto others, is probably finished to you (possibly not on this lifetime, however in the long run). Your purpose is to experience love and satisfaction at the same time as you're right here on Earth. Earth and lifestyles here's a lovely playground. We can create - and do - a few thing we preference. But we need to understand how creation works. And fulfill our soul's mission right proper here on Earth.

Childhood is often what messes us up. We are born into households who do not apprehend us, who abuse us or who abandon us. This causes us to down load faulty programming. Abusive relationships are proof of this faulty programming. And by means of downloading lousy programming from formative years that doesn't serve us (blocks or stops us) we are simply stopping our evolution.

In order to hold to improvement, we want to make certain we smooth out a few difficulty blocking us or preventing us. Like a new pc, we need to be optimised and running fast and efficiently freed from viruses and files that we not want.

One have to argue that through manner of technique of making new varieties of generation we're in truth trying to play God. Technologists can also in fact be growing what we are – looking for to software program program fact (digital reality, augmented truth) and apprehend how our thoughts works (synthetic intelligence) and reflect the biological spacesuit (robots). That is why it's so essential to recognize how we artwork and apprehend how generation works. We need to make certain we are not designing technology an awesome manner to manipulate us, however as an alternative beautify us.

## Chapter 11: What Are Limiting Beliefs?

Limiting ideals are truly beliefs we hooked up about ourselves and our truth to preserve ourselves regular. Please don't experience bad approximately yourself-imposed boundaries. You have been actually looking for to live on.

Beliefs are established as part of your studying software (studies) and presupposed to maintain you secure in unstable or difficult situations on the identical time as you were developing up. But as we grow to be older and begin to create our lives, we bump up in competition to those ideals and they may be able to sometimes be limitations.

Limitations can regularly be placed at the same time as we strive to seem, begin to create a few factor new in our lives or explore a modern area. Often we are met with blocks, sabotage, the equal antique same antique or intense emotional triggers that try to prevent us. This can impair our evolution.

Beliefs are anchored to emotions that lead us to past memories stored in our subconscious. We can get right of entry to those in a hypnotic country and effects delete and re-write the studies to create the high-quality feasible final outcomes.

Like Joe Dispenza always says, in case you want to alternate your life, first you need to alternate your electricity.

How to Identify Limiting Beliefs aka Safety Limits

Since your outer fact is a pondered photograph of your inner reality. To exchange your outer reality, you have to first alternate your internal reality. And the fine place to start is through taking stock of your proscribing beliefs.

Have you ever provide you with a brilliant concept, felt simply energised and inspired after which blasted off to get began and carry out a touch artwork making prepared to transport this new concept into the world even as unexpectedly the voices in your head begin telling you that "you could't do that, you're too terrible, in any other case you're no longer quite sufficient, otherwise you're not certified to try this?"

These little voices are your ego reaffirming your restricting beliefs. The ego serves because the narrator - it's going to tell us some component notion we've got locked into our subconscious.

When we step out of autopilot and start to create our lives, the ones restricting beliefs, with the assist of our trusty ego, try and keep us consistent by blockading us.

We are powerful creators who come right right here to Earth to occur what's internal us. We use the quantum area to bring about what we desire onto the material aircraft. If we aren't growing the existence we need, we're blocked and fixed and most probably developing from a perception device that modified into installation in us with the aid of manner of manner of our mother and father, traumas, society, faith, and masses of others (all the applications walking that aren't authentically us).

To create the lifestyles we need, we must easy and re-write those proscribing beliefs.

A Limiting Belief Story

When I actually have grow to be a infant I preferred to be a health practitioner. I had a clinical doctor's bundle, studied anatomy, understood the way the body labored and pretended to artwork on my teddy bears and dolls. My mother didn't assume that emerge as an super plan. When I emerge as 9, she told me that I have become awful at math and might in no way be capable of get into medical school. Rather than encouraging me to have a look at my dream and assist me emotionally and academically, she helped me software a limiting belief into my unconscious which then come to be severa proscribing ideals. These beliefs were "I'm not clever sufficient. I'm not correct sufficient. I'm awful at math. I can't be who I need. I will by no means get into clinical university and emerge as a systematic health practitioner. I will fail."

Looking back, she have become trying to find to assist me. She believed I want to discover a profession that become tons less complex for me to pursue. But due to what she stated, I gave up on my dream, stopped studying anatomy, stopped healing my teddy bears and dolls and felt misplaced inside the global. I started to fail math and save you making use of myself in school. After nearly failing out of immoderate university, I determined I desired some component better for myself. I enrolled at a community university and changed how I confirmed up at college. I ended up getting the first-rate marks within the college and all A's in my math commands. I went straight away to some other college, obtained an academic scholarship, graduated with honours and function continually used records and information to inform all factors of my life. Now, I paintings based absolutely mostly on what's in alignment with my center values and actual notion device.

My mom had unmarried-handedly re-created my lifestyles's course with one statement based completely totally on her perception system. I took on her belief that I grow to be "awful at math," believed it and made it my truth.

If she had as a substitute stated, "you are having a piece hassle with math right now, and I understand you really need to be a health practitioner, so I will help you observe," my lifestyles must have grew to turn out to be out very in a exceptional way.

Until I became capable of re-write this enjoy and easy my restricting beliefs, I by no means felt like I became strolling in a career that was my authentic calling. I felt like I became absolutely running to get a pay-take a look at and forcing myself to move away my actual self on the door. I end up constantly strolling for narcissistic bosses who did no longer see my fee and attempted to impose their notion structures on me.

These varieties of evaluations show up so regularly in our life that if we without a doubt went again to our youth, we might be surprised at how willing we had been to different human beings shaping our lives. And even as you smooth proscribing beliefs, that's exactly what you need to do.

Once I was capable of clean and re-write the ones restricting ideals, I realised that what I preferred to do have become take a look at vitamins and assist people heal. So I did certainly that with terrific ease and glide.

Many instances the universe will display us that we are on the incorrect direction thru manner of creating matters particularly hard. The more hard and chaotic our existence is, the extra we have strayed from our real self and our divine path.

The Myth of Positive Affirmations

A lot of humans keep in mind that through honestly announcing effective affirmations over and over they'll easy their proscribing ideals. I've in no way positioned this to be the case. Positive affirmations are a first-rate manner to become aware of proscribing ideals, however to reprogram your unconscious you need to head once more to the idea reason of the issue, easy it, re-write it and embody your new creation.

Without going lower lower back to the premise purpose (the revel in/trauma from a long term 0 - 14 that implanted the proscribing notion), the hassle will not be absolutely cleared and re-programmed. But saying effective affirmations is great too – it's just like planting a lawn over a toxic waste sell off. Eventually the ones plant life die until you easy the soil underneath. And your ego may be operating time past law to reveal your subconscious narrative does not in shape what you are saying.

Our Mission Here on Earth

When we incarnate in this lifetime we come right here with a particular challenge. Our project is to unique our real self or our soul's expression and evolve as thousands as we probable can in our lifetime. When we discover, encompass and serve the sector from our soul essence, we gain the right which means that of achievement.

Soul missions (lifestyles reason) range and it is as a lot as you to discover yours. For instance, you will be right proper right here to provide the arena with new track, art work, clinical discoveries, nurturing, splendor, compassion, love - you do not have to come right right here to come to be the subsequent Elon Musk or Barack Obama. Everyone has a unique assignment for each lifetime.

Unfortunately, society has special plans for us. Society takes our undertaking and re-packages it to in form its own assignment (insert what you take delivery of as true with that mission to be here_____ slavery, loss of life, destruction, chaos). And if we want to get decrease returned to our proper self, we should observe what ideals are lurking in our unconscious and re-software program the ones to loose ourselves so we can create the lifestyles we were presupposed to stay.

Examples of Limiting Beliefs

- It's dangerous for me to be myself

- I'm don't have enough time

- That is probably too tough

- Money is evil

- Rich humans are evil

- Money is tough to make

- I'll continuously be broke

- I'll simplest be loved if I human beings-please

- I will get hurt, people will damage me

- Change will kill me

- Life is tough

- I'm now not genuine sufficient

- I'm no longer worth

- I am unfortunate

- I am all on my own, I don't have any assist

- I can be killed/murdered

- I don't want to be happy/wealthy/a achievement

- No one loves me – I am unworthy of love

- Men/Women are evil

- I will fail

- I'm now not regular

- I can't cope with it

- I can't advantage fulfillment

- I am powerless

- I cannot perform a touch trouble

The styles of beliefs are special for all of us and rely upon the testimonies.

All of these beliefs are connected to feelings and research in our lifetime that form us. The trick to reprogramming your unconscious is to determine the horrific patterns in your lifestyles, take a look at what's causing those patterns (it's typically an experience from some time zero – 14) and then clearing and re-writing those critiques to open up your existence to health, happiness and abundance. Following styles, feelings and triggers are a exquisite vicinity to begin investigating your blocks and faulty programming.

What Happens When You Re-Program?

By clearing and re-writing proscribing ideals, you may re-application your inner truth and therefore create an outer reality that resonates and displays your real self. It's like taking the breaks off with reference to dwelling lifestyles on your phrases and manifesting. And whilst you start clearing you become limitless and unstoppable. There isn't some thing we are able to't do!

How do you understand you've effectively re-programmed?

-      you revel in happier, freer and greater accepting

-   what you consciously desire in lifestyles starts offevolved offevolved to expose up

-      you are not emotionally triggered and enjoy courageous and uninhibited

-   you revel in like 'your self'

-   you're non violent and snug in any situation

-   you consider yourself and understand that you may be appropriate enough regardless of what

- lifestyles will become a lovely thriller

- your friends and social circle adjustments to embody happier, more healthy people

- you exchange your focus to living your soul undertaking

- addictions and poisonous behaviours end

- you are taking your fitness notably

- life becomes more harmonious and congruent

- you could effects find out your styles and behaviours that throw you off balance

This is also the foundational center of BELIEF HACKING™

Emotional Regulation & Clearing

Before you learn how to smooth beliefs, first you should get familiar collectively together with your emotions and at the same time as and the way you revel in certain ones. This is an instance of an emotion chart. You can learn how to clean feelings in the Emotional Regulation & Clearing workshop on my website www.Bigbeautifulsky.Com.

Diet & LIfestyle to Heal Trauma

Healing trauma involves taking stock of your emotions, restricting ideals however additionally assisting your self through food plan and workout.

There is an ebook and weight-reduction plan available for every person looking to similarly beautify highbrow and bodily health further to heal trauma I wrote known as Become Limitless™: Optimal Nutrition for Mind-Body-Spirit.

In this ebook you will discover ways to use a researched-backed meals gadget to restore your frame from the mobile diploma. All the recipes are designed to assist the frame restore and run optimally, in particular after strain, trauma/PTSD.

It is also a top notch idea to help your body with vitamins with the useful resource of:

- Taking a daily multivitamin with activated B vitamins

- Taking a day by day dose of remarkable magnesium

- Supporting your gut fitness with excessive brilliant probiotics

- Drinking at the least 3L of water in keeping with day

- Sleeping at the least eight hours consistent with night time

- Exercising for at the least half-hour, 5 days in keeping with week

Removing espresso, chocolate and sugar from your food regimen is important as this will help loosen up your demanding tool. You cannot heal trauma with an excessively activated and dysregulated irritating device.

## Chapter 12: Accessing The Subconscious

Think of your unconscious mind as a huge database that shops everything now not on your aware (analytical) thoughts.

It stores your ideals, testimonies, recollections, capabilities, traumas and everything that you have seen, completed or idea. It is likewise your steering device. Your subconscious video show units the facts coming from the senses and categorize them as risks, possibilities, pleasures, triggers, and so forth. It retrieves that data (primarily based absolutely completely to your perception tool) and communicates that statistics for your conscious thoughts where it's miles processed and interpreted into the triumphing 2nd. I apprehend – how cool!

When we meditate and gradual down our breath, we allow float of the aware thoughts and drop into our subconscious. The subconscious takes over our slowed respiration and we forestall having to even recollect it. As our brains drop into beta, alpha and then theta waves, we fall deeper and deeper into our unconscious. This is likewise what's called the 'quantum location.' It is through our unconscious that we can talk with the universe and get proper of access to now not tremendous beyond statistics but future information as well.

Communicating with our unconscious thoughts is executed via feelings. Emotionally charged mind and critiques right now retrieve information. These feelings can motive a terrible or first rate response – however this all relies upon at the notion this is retrieved. Just so that you understand, the negative feelings are typically more potent than the excellent ones. This is likewise how we 'perception hack' – we take a look at the emotion returned to the idea reason of the event that has trapped a proscribing notion in your subconscious.

For instance, allow's say you really started dating someone. You skip on a few superb dates and you then truly don't pay interest from the individual for some days. You get apprehensive, you want to recognize why. Suddenly, you're prompted emotionally and feeling very horrible about the entire enjoy. Your date texts you day after today and apologises. They've been coping with a sick determine. You in spite of the reality which could't shake the awful feeling no matter the truth that there can be a legitimate, logical reason. Why? Because this event brought on a reminiscence out of your unconscious at the same time as you felt rejected. The notion have become "I'm now not correct sufficient."

Removing terrible beliefs is critical for your ongoing fitness and normal overall performance. Since we create our reality from our unconscious ideals, we need to make certain the beliefs we have got stored in our subconscious are beneficial and powerful.

For instance, if we've got got beliefs locked in that inform us "we are able to in no way be happy," then that is the reality we will create — we can be sad our entire lifetime. If we have ideals locked in that sign "we are cherished and supported," then that's what we are able to create — a lifestyles surrounded thru people who love and useful resource us.

How We Create

Your subconscious thoughts may moreover create primarily based absolutely mostly on preference. Desire has a actually effective price and fuels your unconscious. Desire method, you will perform a little aspect a good way to gain the item of your desire. It furthermore opens all available channels to the conscious thoughts for data on how to do this. This is why people say "look at your ardour" or "have a study your cause." It permits us to tap into choice which receives us obsessed on developing the final outcomes we want.

If you placed your aim and it will become the all-consuming obsession of your life, then you'll be a success. When you have got were given set your subconscious mind at the project sponsored up thru that sturdy emotion, then it would allow you to see the opportunities in life that might lead you in your intention. The well-known "Follow your bliss and doors will open..," tells this particular tale.

Worry and worry also can cause the unconscious into developing a miles much less than relevant final results. Both the ones emotions purpose the combat-or-flight hormone release that shuts down our logical minds and maintains us appearing out of a worse-case-situation. We are likely to create what we fear most if we live centered on the trigger.

If you want to show up your choice, then the fantastic way to achieve this is to entwine it with purpose, love, faith and bodily praise (sex as an example). This is why visualisation throughout meditation is so critical. If you could create your preferred final consequences in the 'quantum subject' your subconscious receives implanted with what you want to create. If you envision this final results frequently, then it's going to seem inside the bodily aircraft and come to be your fact.

Brain Waves

As adults, we spend most of our time in conscious mind beta waves. We are busy processing facts from the outer international, studying it, and storing it. When we turn out to be comfortable, our mind-waves drop into low-variety beta. Reading a e-book is an instance.

When we're in a rustic of centered interest, our thoughts-waves drop into mid-range beta. When we're in fight-or-flight, our body produces stress hormones, and launches into excessive-variety beta. It's widespread chaos.

We input alpha range in the course of the number one levels of meditation. By certainly final our eyes and that specialize in our breath, we lessen the records stepping into our mind via eighty%. We study heaps less and start to revel in comfortable. If we preserve focusing inwards inside the route of meditation, then our thoughts-waves sluggish down even in addition and enter into theta variety.

During theta, we are capable to speak with our unconscious. Here we are able to re-software program, take away limiting beliefs and actively visualise what we choice. This is why a success marketers meditate – it's in our subconscious that we get admission to the records we need to obtain.

If we take note of our instinct and often visit our subconscious, then we've got all the solutions. We are our personal courses. That is why the antique announcing "the whole lot you need is positioned internal you" rings real. It clearly is.

## Chapter 13: Discovering Our True Selves

Now that we aren't trapped in a violent relationship, it is time to get again to being ourselves. Be egocentric. Love your self. Treat yourself so kindly. Be your remarkable buddy and your maximum dedicated advise. Back your self.

Don't apprehend wherein to begin? Don't truly apprehend who you are anymore?

Start with some inner little one paintings. Who had been you while you had been little? Who did you want to be? What did you love doing? What did you dream approximately experiencing? What did you faux to be? Who were you friends and why did you want them?

It's also a high-quality idea to find out some structures at the side of:

Astrology - Soul Blueprint (why you are here and your soul undertaking in this life)

Human Design - How You Manifest/ Co-Create

Myers Briggs - Communication Style

DeMartini Value Determination Process - Helps you grow to be aware about your values for alignment

Join groups and flow into find amusing! Dance and rejoice your freedom. This is your danger to begin smooth. Be courageous and be seen!

Clearing Old Energy

Welcome in your sparkling begin. From proper right here it's far critical to keep subjects shifting. Make certain you clear your energy similarly to the energy in your home. You can't circulate on in case you're sitting within the identical electricity day in and time out. Here are a few guidelines for transferring on:

1. Get divorced. Make tremendous you get the papers signed!

2. Change your closing name. If you have the equal name as your abuser, change it as fast as viable. Claim yourself.

three. Remove any momentos or bodily items from your home that remind you of your abuser. If you don't want to throw it away, as a minimum placed it away so you aren't reminded.

four. Keep open-minded. If it is on your pleasant interest to move to a new residence, metropolis,

metropolis, state, u . S . A . To start sparkling - DO IT!

five. Take care of your bodily fitness: consume healthy, glowing meals; exercise; relaxation and lighten up.

6. Meet new pals: exit and see how many new humans you could meet (do now not stay in the past - do not blame or talk on and on about what befell to you).

7. Open yourself as much as new opportunities: discover a new assignment, be part of organizations and studies new talents

8. Be excessive satisfactory to keep slicing energetic cords among yourself and your abuser.

9. Always be honest together together together with your children. Just inform them the reality and do now not communicate badly approximately the opposite determine.

10. Most importantly do what works for you. Only make picks which can be to your super interest.

Find Your ACE Score (click on on on right right here). This will tell how a first rate deal trauma you professional as a little one and what type of recovery is needed.

The records has confirmed that the primary manner to defeat weather trade is to empower women and girls.

Domestic violence is a microcosm of what's taking place inside the complete international (macrocosm). The violence and abuse we enjoy in our non-public houses is happening all around the global to billions of people in a whole lot of strategies.

When we heal ourselves, we unfastened up ourselves and alternate the frequency of not handiest ourselves, but the entire planet (universe). When we heal ourselves we're able to then assist others heal.

"It is not viable to enslave a person who lives with fact in their private strength, liberated from worry and loving of the self."

- Dylan Charles

## Chapter 14: The Workbook

To get the most from this workbook, please solution all the questions and journaling activates. Answering one in step with day is the awesome way to method this magazine. Give yourself time to mirror and be honest.

There isn't any higher way to determine the way you sincerely feel until you write all of it down. You can print this ebook or you may simply answer all the activates on your personal mag.

Please additionally make sure this information is regular from your abuser. If you do not have a secure location to write down down down and mirror please wait until you do. Safety want to continually be your first priority.

The goal of this workbook is to help you understand who you're, what you're experiencing, how you're feeling, why you created your contemporary lifestyles and what you absolutely want to create and enjoy inside the destiny.

Domestic violence and abuse appears like a prison. But you have the vital factor to break out.

You normally did. And now it is time to launch the chains and fly.

Always recognize that your existence is treasured, which you are unique and your enjoy proper here on Earth is needed. Nothing isn't feasible and you are more effective and resilient than you may recognize.

If ever dubious, caught in worry or intend to self-damage, please attain out for help. The international is whole of people who have been within the equal vicinity you've got got and apprehend the way out. You are in no way alone. We are all right proper right here for you and cannot wait to appearance the exceptional new existence you create.

Lots of affection,

Christina

1. What's your tale?

Write down your narrative.

Tell your tale.

Let pass of your conscious thoughts and allow your hands tell the story.

This is referred to as computerized writing.

You'd be amazed what emerges at the same time as you start to piece together the recollections that make up your life.

Use a journal or crack open your laptop and write all of it out.

Where have been you born?

What have become your youth like?

Who have been your mother and father?

What took place to you at the identical time as you have been growing up?

Highlights?

Traumas?

Who cherished you the maximum?

Who abused you?

How does your hero/heroine adventure begin and surrender?

2. Radical Responsibility

What are some of the techniques you can take radical responsibility for your existence? List them proper here:

How does it feel to take radical duty for your existence?

How will subjects alternate even as you are taking radical obligation?

three. How did you experience abuse?

Get honest with yourself.

Understanding the kinds of abuse and the way they have been used to manipulate you is an important step in stopping further abuse.

Now write down all the tactics that abuse made you sense. LIST IT ALL (it's well enough to sense anger, disgrace and grow to be enraged - it's critical to perceive your feelings and set them free).

What are the opportunity emotions to those feelings? Identify the way you'd need to sense as a substitute. These feelings is probably your new north movie star.

four. Dispelling Gaslighting

Can you really come to be aware about gaslighting?

How emerge as gaslighting utilized in opposition to you?

How did it make you revel in?

Do you accept as actual with yourself?

List the methods you still doubt yourself.

What are a few techniques you could start to pay attention to your instinct again?

What does reality propose to you?

How will having truth on your existence alternate matters?

5. People You Trust

Who are you capable of open up to approximately your abusive relationship?

Who are you capable of accumulate out to for assist leaving?

What offerings are to be had to help you transition from your situation?

Who will help you resolve the years of abuse/trauma?

Who permit you to with the care of your youngsters or a few different dependents?

How does it sense to undergo in thoughts?

How will having hold in mind for your life trade things for you?

6. Putting Yourself First

List all the strategies you placed distinctive humans first.

Now list all of the processes you need to begin putting your self first.

How does this make you experience?

How will your life be tremendous when you start putting yourself first?

7. Setting Boundaries

What forms of barriers do you want to installation to guard your self? Remember, limitations are the manner you show humans the way you want to be handled.

Some examples of limitations encompass:

- If you abuse me, I will name the police and report your behavior.

- You cannot go through my subjects without my permission (this consists of chests of drawers, closets, desks, journals, laptop structures, social media and distinctive payments).

- You have to continuously speak to me in a deferential way and tone.

- It's good enough for me to spend as lots time as I would really like with friends and own family.

- I need as an lousy lot time as I'd need to go to the gymnasium, purchase glowing food, go to the physician and carry out unique forms of self-care.

- I will always have my private monetary institution account which you may not have access to.

- I do now not need my personal data shared with different people without my permission

How does it enjoy to have barriers in your existence?

How will your lifestyles alternate when you have limitations for your existence?

8. Saying NO

Who are all the human beings you need to have a look at to say NO to?

What are all of the belongings you need to save you doing?

How will pronouncing NO set you free?

How will it feel to say NO?

How will your existence trade while you are saying NO?

nine. Self-Care

List all the approaches you want to start searching after yourself.

Make time each week to ensure you're showing your self which you are as critical as absolutely everyone else.

Do you need help to make sure you meet yourself-care dreams? If so, please listing who will let you whilst you cope with yourself.

How will having greater self-care in your existence make you revel in?

How will focusing on self-care change your life?

10. Critical Inner Voices

What are some of the vital stuff you say to your self?

Who does your internal voice sound like?

Does it remind you of someone (it's commonly a family member)?

What are a few strategies you could start to apprehend this inner critic and begin to silence it?

How will it sense to disregard your critical internal voice?

How will your existence change while you learn how to overlook about your internal critic?

eleven. Investing in Yourself

What are a few competencies you want to observe?

Are there schooling you would really like to take?

Music/performs/films you need to look?

Bucket list gadgets you want to tick off? Now is the time to do YOU!

How does it experience to put money into yourself?

How will your life exchange even as you spend money on your self?

12. Toxic People

Who in your life drains you, makes you experience horrific approximately yourself, reasons drama or gossips/puts others down?

Make a listing after which set up company boundaries spherical how they could act for your presence.

Do you want to eliminate them out of your life certainly? You decide what's excellent for you.

How will it revel in to cast off toxic human beings from your life?

How will your life alternate as soon as these people aren't on your life?

thirteen. Codependency

How are you sacrificing your self for others?

In what strategies do you positioned others first rather than yourself?

Do you resent each person on your lifestyles?

If so, is it due to the fact you're giving manner an excessive amount of to them and no longer enough to yourself? Change that. Write down how you intend to make certain you break the dependancy of codependency.

How will it feel to position your self first?

How will your existence exchange whilst you do?

14. Trauma

Are you experiencing any physical symptoms and signs and signs and symptoms out of your abuse which incorporates autoimmune troubles, thyroid problems, tension or despair?

List some thing you observed might be attributed or associated on your trauma.

Trauma furthermore shows up in our relationships. Do your relationships mirror your relationships to primary caregivers?

Feel into your frame. Where do you feel you maintain maximum of your emotions? Be high-quality to stretch and supply your frame love.

## 15. Emotions

When you feel compelled, disturbing and taken about what feelings do you revel in?

Do those emotions remind you of conditions from youth (a while zero-7)?

Can you operate mindfulness (gift 2d) and breathwork to calm your self?

What are wholesome techniques to preserve yourself from spiraling right right into a delivered on state? List them.

Do you permit your self sense and express your emotions? If not, how will you start to exchange that now?

## 16. Limiting Beliefs

List the strategies you limit yourself.

Can you listen your internal critic?

What does he/she say whilst you want to strive some thing new?

How do you keep your self lower back?

What issue does worry play in your existence?

How will it feel to live limitlessly?

How will your lifestyles alternate whilst you begin to live limitlessly?

17. True Self

What are some subjects you can do to discover your proper self?

What are some pursuits you may start for you to "fill you up?"

Where are the humans you want to fulfill?

What places have you ever been searching for to go to?

Start tuning in to what you absolutely desire. This is your self talking to you.

How will it revel in to stay as your real self?

How will your lifestyles exchange while you live your life as your actual self?

18. New Life

What does your new life appear to be? Write down precisely what you need to enjoy, how it will experience and what you need to do to perform that. Dream BIG! And enjoy how it would experience to live YOUR AMAZING NEW LIFE. And then take movement to create it.

Part I: Child Abuse

Child abuse continues to stand up at exquisite costs in U.S. Society. Nearly 1½ % of youngsters have been sufferers of toddler abuse in a unmarried three hundred and sixty five days (2008). Approximately seventy two% of them professional overlook, 16% had been physical abused, 9% were sexually abused, and 7% had been psychologically/emotionally abused. More than half of these kids have been underneath eight years of age (Rubin, 2012, p. Three). Disturbing as the ones numbers are, they likely represent handiest the stop of the iceberg. Not all incidents of abuse are said or substantiated. The actual incidence of infant maltreatment is a wonderful deal better than the substantiated price.

Finkelhor et al. (2005) anticipated that one in seven, or nearly 15% of youths are maltreated in the long run in adolescence or early life. The range of unreported times is a long way extra, because of the reality the youngsters are afraid to tell everyone what has passed off, and the jail methods for validating an episode can be difficult. The lengthy-term emotional and mental damage of physical and/or sexual abuse can be devastating to the kid. The problem wants to be identified, the abuse stopped, and the kid and circle of relatives offered expert assist.

Child abuse can take area in the family, through a discern, stepparent, sibling or extraordinary relative; or out of doors the residence, for example, with the resource of using a friend, neighbor, childcare man or woman, teacher, or stranger. When abuse has occurred, a infant can boom a number of distressing emotions, thoughts and behaviors.

A Historical Perspective

The American Academy of Child and Adolescent Psychiatry publishes exercising parameters for the forensic evaluation of youngsters and more youthful those who may also moreover had been physically or sexually abused (AACAP, 1997, or see www.Aacap.Org). In the parameters is this short records of the recognition of infant abuse.

In the 1860s, a French forensic pathologist defined the battered-infant syndrome after appearing autopsies on kids who've been crushed to loss of life (Tardieu, 1860, 1868). In america, little one abuse got here to public interest thru the case of Mary Ellen, an 8-three hundred and sixty five days-antique girl who modified into severely maltreated (Ross, 1977). She become placed through church humans in New York City in 1874, but they placed that the tremendous organisation that modified into to be had to assist became the Society for the Prevention of Cruelty to Animals. Thus, they founded The Society for the Prevention of Cruelty to Children. In 1875, New York changed into the number one country to adopt a baby safety regulation, which have come to be the model for tremendous states.

In the 20 th century, the rediscovery of child abuse modified into signaled thru the use of a radiologist in a sanatorium emergency room. Caffey (1946) observed a syndrome of children with a couple of skeletal injuries and chronic subdural hematomas. Up till the Nineteen Sixties, it turned into idea that bodily abuse of children end up uncommon--partly due to the reality bodily problem of children changed into typically extra relevant and in component because of societal denial regarding violence within the route of children. In an vital article within the Journal of the American Medical Association, Kempe et al. (1962) defined the battered-little one syndrome. In 1974 the federal government surpassed the Child Abuse Prevention and Treatment Act, which led to each state passing jail hints in which targeted people were required to record infant abuse.

Definitions of Terms

Definitions of various sides of home violence and the legally mandated responses are decided with the beneficial resource of every nation, however federal law offers a basis for states thru the usage of identifying a tough and speedy of acts or behaviors that define abuse. For example, the Child Abuse Prevention and Treatment Act (CAPTA), (forty U.S.C. §5101), as amended by way of way of the CAPTA Reauthorization Act of 2010 (CAPTA, 2010), offers the following definition of infant abuse and neglect approximately:

Any current act or failure to behave at the a part of a determine or caretaker which leads to dying, vital bodily or emotional harm, sexual abuse or exploitation; or an act or failure to behave, which offers an drawing close risk of first-rate damage.

Each u . S . A . Is responsible for imparting its very private definitions of toddler abuse and overlook about in the civil and criminal codes. Civil statutes describe the occasions and conditions that obligate mandated journalists to file said or suspected times of abuse, and that they provide definitions critical for juvenile/circle of relatives courts power of mind of toddler dependency. Criminal statutes specify the kinds of maltreatment which might be criminally punishable.

The Federal Child Abuse Prevention and Treatment Act (CAPTA), amended and reauthorized in 2010, gives the following definitions:

Child is someone who has no longer attained the lesser of:

• The age of 18; or

• Except in instances of sexual abuse, the age unique thru the child protection law of the State wherein the child is living.

Child abuse and overlook is, at a minimum:

• Any current-day act or failure to behave at the a part of a discern or caretaker which results in loss of life, severe bodily or emotional damage, sexual abuse or exploitation; or

• An act or failure to act which offers an coming near near risk of super harm.

Sexual abuse is:

• The employment, use, persuasion, inducement, enticement, or coercion of any baby to have interaction in, or help another character to interact in, any sexually unique conduct or simulation of such conduct for the purpose of manufacturing a seen depiction of such conduct; or

• The rape, and in instances of caretaker or inter-familial relationships, statutory rape, molestation, prostitution, or one-of-a-kind shape of sexual exploitation of children, or incest with kids.

Source:

http://www.Acf.Hhs.Gov/programs/cb/laws_polic
ies/cblaws/capta/capta2010.Pdf

Bullying

Another elegance of abuse that need to no longer
be neglected is bullying, described in reality as
"using aggression to harm a few other individual"
(Fife and Schrager, 2012, p. 45). Bullying typically
takes place at faculty, and might encompass
emotional aggression, which include name-calling
and exclusion from corporations.

According to Fife and Schrager, bullying does no
longer take place in a vacuum, but can amplify
past the bully and the bullied to special
youngsters, who are aware about it and can
forget approximately approximately or maybe
help and resource the bullying. Teachers and
different adults can be at least in element aware
of what is going on however do now not
intervene. Certain children may be at higher risk
of being bullied via using virtue of being first-rate
in some manner. For example, kids can be much
more likely to be bullied if they may be: new at
faculty, obese, not on time or disabled and/or
gay.

A present day-day extension of the concept is cyber-bullying, in which the competitive behaviors can amplify to harassment via virtual conversation media like e-mail, texting, and social networking web sites. According to the CDC e-book Electronic Media and Youth Violence (Hertz and David-Ferdon, 2008), "Electronic Aggression is any kind of harassment or bullying (teasing, telling lies, making a laugh of someone, making impolite or endorse remarks, spreading rumors, or making threatening or aggressive comments) that takes area via electronic mail, a talk room, on the spot messaging, a internet internet web page (together with blogs), or text messaging."

How commonplace is virtual aggression? Because it's far a cutting-edge phenomenon and due to the fact exclusive researchers have used differing terminology to explain and description it, we have very limited proof-primarily based absolutely statistics. Hertz and David-Ferdon (2008) predicted that approximately nine% to 35% of more youthful human beings say they were the victim of digital aggression. (Fife and Schrager, 2012, p. Forty seven) expected the prevalence of cyber-bullying amongst 23% and seventy two% amongst middle and high college students. The differing fees and huge levels are attributed to the early america of research in this place.

Not distinctly, digital aggression is becoming more common. According to Hertz and David-Ferdon (2008) "In 2000, 6% of net clients a long term 10-17 stated they were the victim of 'on line harassment,' described as threats or other offensive conduct [not sexual solicitation] sent online to someone or published on line. By 2005, this percentage had expanded via 50%, to nine%. As generation will become more much less highly-priced and complicated, fees of digital aggression are probably to preserve to increase, especially if suitable prevention and intervention tips and practices aren't positioned into area."

What troubles are associated with virtual aggression? Once once more, there are as but few managed studies, but a number of the consequences that have been identified (Hertz and David-Ferdon, 2008) are:

• alcohol and drug use

• school detentions or suspensions

• college absences

• in-individual victimization

Numbers of Victims of Child Abuse

The following records are from the National Child Abuse and Neglect Data System (NCANDS) document Child Maltreatment 2010 (US DHHS, 2010). During Federal economic 12 months 2010, an predicted three.Three million referrals, related to the alleged maltreatment of about five.Nine million children, had been acquired by CPS groups. The victim fee come to be 695,000 (9.2 sufferers in step with 1,000) children inside the population.

Sadly, youngsters more youthful than 1 yr of age had the satisfactory rate of victimization at 20.6 in step with 1,000 youngsters within the population of the identical age. Victims with the single-12 months age of one, 2, or three years antique had victimization quotes of eleven.Nine, 11.Four, and 11.Zero victims in keeping with 1,000 kids of those respective a while inside the populace. In modern, the price and percent of victimization decreased with age.

Victimization have become cut up among the sexes, with boys accounting for forty eight.Five percentage and girls accounting for 51.2 percentage. Less than 1 percent of victims had an unknown sex.

Eighty-eight percentage of unique sufferers have been constructed from three races or ethnicities—African-American, Hispanic, and White. However, sufferers of African-American, more than one racial descents, and American Indian or Alaska Native had the very nice fees of victimization at 14.6, 12.7, and 11.Zero patients, respectively, in keeping with 1,000 children in the populace of the identical race or ethnicity.

As in preceding years, the satisfactory chances of kids were not noted. A toddler can also have suffered from a couple of varieties of maltreatment and have become counted as soon as for every maltreatment type. CPS investigations or tests decided that for specific patients:

• More than 75 percentage (seventy eight.Three%) suffered neglect approximately

• More than 15 percentage (17.6%) suffered bodily abuse

• Less than 10 percentage (9.2%) suffered sexual abuse

Child fatalities are the maximum tragic very last results of maltreatment. Yet, every 365 days children die from abuse and forget about about. Fifty-one States said a total of one,537 fatalities. Based on these data, a nationally anticipated 1,560 children died from abuse and overlook. Analyses are achieved on the form of infant fatalities for whom case-diploma facts had been received. Of the stated fatalities:

• The standard fee of toddler fatalities became 2.07 deaths regular with a hundred,000 kids.

• Boys had a better toddler fatality rate than women at 2.Fifty one boys in keeping with a hundred,000 boys within the populace.

• Girls died of abuse and forget at a fee of one.Seventy 3 consistent with one hundred,000 ladies inside the population.

• Nearly eighty percent (79.4%) of all infant fatalities were younger than four years antique.

• More than 40 percentage (40.8%) of toddler fatalities had been because of a couple of maltreatment sorts.

• More than 30 percentage (32.6%) of toddler fatalities have been attributed absolutely to neglect.

Risk elements for little one abuse and forget embody the following (tailored from Fife and Schrager, 2012, p. 31):

• Younger age of the mom

• Maternal depression or substance abuse

• Single-figure circle of relatives

• Poverty

• Households wherein intimate accomplice violence takes vicinity

Who Abused and Neglected Children?

For the analyses blanketed in this report (National Child Abuse and Neglect Data System (NCANDS) document Child Maltreatment 2010 (US DHHS, 2010), a perpetrator is the individual that is responsible for the abuse or forget about approximately of a little one. Fifty States cautioned case-stage data about perpetrators the use of particular identifiers. In those States, the complete unique rely quantity of perpetrators changed into 510,824. For 2010:

• Four-fifths (eighty one.Three%) of sufferers were maltreated by using way of a discern either appearing by myself or with a person else.

• One-fifth (18.Five%) of patients have been maltreated with the aid of the usage of method of every dad and mom.

• Nearly -fifths (37.2%) of sufferers had been maltreated thru their mother acting on my own.

• One-fifth (19.1%) of sufferers have been maltreated via their father acting on my own.

• Thirteen percent of sufferers were maltreated with the useful resource of a perpetrator who modified into not a decide of the child.

• More than -fifths (45.2%) of perpetrators have been men and multiple-half of (53.6%) were women.

• More than one-0.33 (36.Three%) of perpetrators were within the age commercial enterprise organisation of 20-29 years.

• More than eighty percent (80 4.2%) of perpetrators had been a number of the a long time of 20 and forty nine years.

The racial distributions of unique perpetrators were much like the race in their sufferers. During FFY 2010, one-half (forty 9.2%) have been White, one-fifth (20.Zero%) of perpetrators were African-American, and one-5th (19.Zero%) of perpetrators had been Hispanic. Race or ethnicity changed into now not endorsed for eight.Five percent of perpetrators. American Indian or Alaska Native, Asian, and multiple race descent accounted for three percent of perpetrators. These proportions have remained regular for the past few years (US DHHS, 2010).

Do Abused Children Become Abusers?

Studies have attempted to discover whether or not or now not youngsters who are abused are much more likely than other kids to emerge as abusers themselves. For example, Hall (2011), in an exploration of the concept of the intergenerational transmission of family violence, cites research suggesting that there can be some of mechanisms wherein youngsters can studies dysfunctional behaviors and express them within the route in their lives. Stated in terms of attachment concept, the abused toddler learns unfavorable dating patterns with an abusive caregiver that can form a template for future relationships. According to Cares (2009), the kid who has been abused develops a disorganized attachment style to adapt to dysfunctional parental bonds and later has trouble altering such patterns. In terms of social gaining knowledge of principle, abused youngsters examine of their families of basis that violent or coercive forms of conduct are profitable – or at the least powerful – so they repeat the pattern in person life.

The concept of intergenerational transmission of circle of relatives violence want to be regarded with caution. First, it's far very important for abused children to avoid developing the expectation that they'll be sure to copy information. Second, there's no dependable empirical consensus in assist of the idea that youngsters who're abused are likely to become abusers. As Hall (2011) warns, "Although there's empirical records that parents who've been abused have better expenses of abusing their personal kids, the idea that family violence can be right now related to abuse inside the next generation has end up arguable because definitions of abuse and costs of reporting are inconsistent and methodological stressful situations for little one abuse research abound…. My studies indicates that there can be gaps in those theories….. Some children may also moreover moreover analyze no longer to do some component they that they see is risky or vain." Hall advocates moving to a strengths-based framework of intervention that locations the point of interest of remedy on person abilities on the way to deliver individuals the opportunity to avoid repeating dysfunctional patterns.

Clinical Screening Procedures to Identify Victims and Perpetrators

Regardless of the facts said above, it is vital that highbrow healthcare providers admire the capability for any infant to be a sufferer and any person to be a wrongdoer (Fife and Schrager, 2012, p. 30). There isn't any sufferer or wrongdoer profile that would characteristic a dependable predictor of chance for any given little one. In different words, there may be no clean regularly taking place presentation of kids who've been abused. Abused kids display up diverse symptoms, a whole lot of emotional, behavioral, and somatic reactions. These signs and symptoms are neither unique nor pathognomonic, in that the same symptoms can also additionally get up with none records of abuse. The signs and symptoms and signs manifested through abused youngsters may be organized into clinical patterns. Although it may be useful to look at whether or not or now not or now not a selected case falls into this kind of patterns that is not in itself diagnostic of infant abuse.

Some of the techniques wherein violent victimization affects children had been stated with the resource of Murphy (2007):

• posttraumatic strain disorder

• aggression

• depression

• issues in social interactions, which include intimate relationships

• lower ranges of educational achievement

• internalization of emotions

Clinical screening strategies to pick out out patients and perpetrators ought to be routinized as part of beginning the evaluation approach at the very onset of treatment. In special terms, the opportunity of abuse or overlook need to be quietly taken into consideration as a capability correlate of the offering symptoms and signs, irrespective of inadvertent or advertent tries at the part of clients to cowl or disavow any such relationship. Child customers can be fearful of disclosing abuse, and their caretakers may be collusive with an abuser.

Initial screening can also include observations of the subsequent signs and symptoms and signs and symptoms and symptoms which can sign the presence of little one abuse or forget (tailor-crafted from the Child Welfare Information Gateway, available at: www.Childwelfare.Gov/pubs/factsheets/signs and symptoms.Cfm):

The Child:

• Shows unexpected changes in behavior or faculty general performance

• Has no longer acquired assist for bodily or medical troubles introduced to the parents' interest

• Has learning issues (or difficulty concentrating) that can not be attributed to precise physical or intellectual causes

• Is typically watchful, as regardless of the truth that getting ready for a few component awful to take region

• Lacks person supervision

• Is overly compliant, passive, or withdrawn

• Comes to school or specific sports early, stays overdue, and does not need to move home

The Parent:

• Shows little undertaking for the kid

• Denies the life of—or blames the child for—the children's problems in university or at home

• Asks instructors or one in all a type caregivers to use harsh physical problem if the kid misbehaves

• Sees the child as definitely terrible, nugatory, or burdensome

• Demands a diploma of bodily or academic common normal performance the child cannot achieve

• Looks commonly to the child for care, attention, and pride of emotional needs

The Parent and Child:

• Rarely contact or study each distinct

• Consider their dating totally horrible

• State that they do now not like each distinct

Types of Abuse

The following are a few symptoms frequently related to unique varieties of little one abuse: physical abuse, overlook about, sexual abuse, and emotional abuse. It is crucial to word, but, that those varieties of abuse are more usually determined in combination than by myself. A physical abused infant, as an instance, is often emotionally abused as properly, and a sexually abused toddler furthermore can be unnoticed.

Consider the possibility of bodily abuse whilst the child:

• Has unexplained burns, bites, bruises, broken bones, or black eyes

• Has fading bruises or unique marks amazing after an absence from college

• Seems afraid of the dad and mom and protests or cries even as it's time to transport home

• Shrinks at the technique of adults

• Reports harm with the aid of manner of a determine or every other individual caregiver

Consider the opportunity of bodily abuse whilst the discern or other individual caregiver:

• Offers conflicting, unconvincing, or no reason behind the children's damage

• Describes the child as "evil," or in some unique very terrible way

• Uses harsh bodily area with the child

• Has a history of abuse as a toddler

Consider the opportunity of neglect whilst the child:

• Is regularly absent from faculty

• Begs or steals meals or cash

• Lacks desired clinical or dental care, immunizations, or glasses

• Is continuously dirty and has extreme frame fragrance

• Lacks sufficient apparel for the climate

• Abuses alcohol or specific capsules

• States that there's no man or woman at home to provide care

Consider the possibility of forget about at the same time as the figure or distinct man or woman caregiver:

• Appears to be detached to the kid

• Seems apathetic or depressed

• Behaves irrationally or in a weird way

• Is abusing alcohol or other drugs

Consider the possibility of sexual abuse while the child:

• Has difficulty taking walks or sitting

• Suddenly refuses to exchange for gym or to participate in bodily sports activities

• Reports nightmares or bedwetting

• Experiences a surprising change in urge for meals

• Demonstrates bizarre, trendy, or unusual sexual data or behavior

• Becomes pregnant or contracts a venereal sickness, in particular if underneath age 14

• Runs away

• Reports sexual abuse by means of the usage of a decide or a few unique person caregiver

Consider the possibility of sexual abuse even as the discern or different person caregiver:

• Is unduly shielding of the kid or severely limits the child's touch with specific kids, specifically of the opposite intercourse

• Is secretive and remoted

• Is jealous or controlling with circle of relatives individuals

Consider the opportunity of emotional maltreatment even as the child:

• Shows extremes in behavior, which includes overly compliant or stressful behavior, extreme passivity, or aggression

• Is every inappropriately person (parenting unique kids, for instance) or inappropriately childish (often rocking or head-banging, as an instance)

• Is not on time in bodily or emotional improvement

• Has attempted suicide

• Reports a loss of attachment to the determine

Consider the opportunity of emotional maltreatment at the same time as the determine or other character caregiver:

• Constantly blames, belittles, or berates the child

• Is unconcerned approximately the kid and refuses to bear in thoughts offers of help for the children's problems

• Overtly rejects the child

Mandatory Reporting of Child Maltreatment

All 50 states, the District of Columbia, Puerto Rico, and the united states territories have criminal recommendations that mandate reporting of toddler maltreatment. Some states use greater particular definitions of who's a mandated reporter. Others pick out greater flexible verbiage is order to strong a wider internet. In all states, healthcare businesses are mandated reporters. In addition, all obligatory reporting crook recommendations use deliberately indistinct descriptors of the quantity of issue or truth the reporter must have in case you need to initiate a document. Some prison guidelines specify "cause to consider…" or "suspect…" so you can gain the brink for reporting. In order to inspire wider compliance, all compulsory crook suggestions embody nicely faith exemptions from civil prosecution if it is ultimately decided that maltreatment can not be substantiated.

In the State of Florida, a present day law took impact on October 1, 2012 that end up touted because the toughest inside the united states of america, called the "Protection of Vulnerable Persons Act." It goes a long way past in advance prison recommendations, which required reporting handiest at the identical time because the suspected abuser turned into a figure or caretaker. For the number one time, the modern law makes reporting of toddler-on-infant abuse compulsory. It applies to any abuser, even folks that are youngsters themselves. Children 12 and beneath who are deemed perpetrators can be referred for treatment and treatment, but the ones 13 and up may be stated law enforcement. Individuals who fail to document abuse and neglect face crook prosecution and fines as much as $five,000.

Coming within the wake of the Penn State scandal, the modern day law additionally stipulates that faculties and universities that "knowingly and willfully" fail to document suspected little one abuse, abandonment or overlook — or save you another person from doing so — now face fines of as a good deal as $1 million for each incident.

Florida hotline numbers and reporting hints can be decided on-line at:

http://www.Dcf.State.Fl.Us/programs/abuse/

For one-of-a-kind states, please talk to the Child Welfare Information Gateway record: Mandatory Reporters of Child Abuse and Neglect: Summary of State Laws, which may be found on-line at:

http://www.Childwelfare.Gov/systemwide/laws_policies/statutes/manda.Cfm

See Appendix A at the end of this course for referral and assets for toddler abuse situations.

Interventions for Victims of Child Abuse

Once a little one protecting offerings file is filed, the therapist might also furthermore now not have the opportunity of strolling with the family. However, in instances wherein therapists do art work with children and households who've prolonged beyond thru the prison infant protection strategies, there are some of evaluation and remedy troubles to be stated.

First, a miles greater entire evaluation need to precede any treatment making plans. According to the Comprehensive Family Assessment

Guidelines for Child Welfare (Schene, 2005), as quickly as infant safety offerings had been put into location, the therapist have to "short glide beyond investigating facts to expand an data of what has took place, including why it has took place and what is going to be required to restore the family's functioning and prevent the recurrence of abuse or forget about. If a family's functioning may be restored, the family can efficiently stay at the coronary heart of the kid's global."

For the competencies of such an assessment, "complete" way that the assessment includes data gathered via each other checks and addresses the wider wishes of the kid and family which could have an effect on a infant's safety, permanency, and nicely-being, in other phrases – the "big photo" – now not simply a hard and rapid of signs and signs and symptoms.

Sample questions that might be asked consist of the following (tailor-made from Schene, 2005):

• What is the proper nature of the abuse and/or forget?

• For how lengthy has the abuse and/or neglect passed off, and what has been the impact on the kid's functioning and development?

• How do the mother and father and the kids view their modern-day scenario?

• What in the dad and mom' beyond and current reviews contributes to the family's needs and issues?

• In what techniques have the mother and father very well provided for his or her kids and what are their strengths?

• What preceding efforts were made with the aid of the dad and mom to fulfill the kid or younger people's goals and remedy the family's issues?

• What kinship assets are available, which includes assets of the tribe or extended family to which the circle of relatives belongs?

• What specific offerings are desired thru the kid and the child's parents to solve the problems which might be requiring defensive offerings?

These questions show that the focal point of a complete own family evaluation isn't only a picture of the imparting problems at a particular time, however moreover a dynamic assessment of the underlying causal factors for behaviors and situations affecting kids. It also consists of evaluation of contributing factors which incorporates own family facts, home violence, substance abuse, highbrow health, continual fitness issues, and poverty. In addition, the circle of relatives's strengths and protecting factors are assessed to perceive assets which could help the own family's capability to fulfill its dreams and higher defend the youngsters.

Consideration of a Strengths-Based Model of Assessment and Treatment

Conventional little one abuse remedy packages often depend on a deficits-based model, wherein parenting deficits and toddler pathology are the point of interest. In a strengths-based totally sincerely model, exquisite psychology offers an asset-based completely model in which capabilities are emphasised and the strengths of the kid and the dad and mom are identified as number one resources. This does not suggest ignoring actual troubles; as an alternative, it way giving greater weight to human beings's strengths and growing opportunities for them to find out their non-public capacities. Positive interventions for abused youngsters and their dad and mom may be specially effective due to the reality both determine and infant are at a aspect at which they may be specially inspired inside the course of alternate (Hall, 2011). The assessment manner have to, then, encompass a detailed survey of sensible property (of the kid and the figure) that will become the premise for intervention.

Some of the circle of relatives's assets/protecting factors that must be explored and implemented in remedy are the following (tailor-made from Schene, 2005):

• Presence of a supportive extended circle of relatives willing and able to assist

• Demonstrated capability of dad and mom to accept obligation for their behavior and willingness to exchange

• Value located on the position of determine and desire to do an top notch undertaking

• Clear knowledge of kids's and little one's developmental desires

• Willingness to fulfill the needs of the kid or young adults; ability to get the child to highschool, medical appointments, and so forth.

• Adjusting region to diploma of development

• Ability to govern expression of anger

• Physical and emotional fitness of figure or caregiver

• Capacity to shape and maintain healthful relationships

• Positive styles of problem solving in one-of-a-kind lifestyles regions

• Parental past revel in protecting the child

• Non-maltreating parent or extraordinary person within the home willing and able to shield the kid

• Appropriate communique and hassle fixing competencies of the adults that share little one care

Treatment

Building at the idea of a strengths-primarily based version brought above, own family remedy may need to minimally comprise the subsequent components (tailored from Hall, 2011):

• Creating safety for the kid or children

• Improving parenting abilties and self-photograph

• Becoming an endorse for the kid

• Seeking social assist for each decide and infant

• Finding role models

• Developing interactive parenting

Although there may be a few not unusual troubles decided among households who have encountered the kid welfare tool (for instance, substance abuse, intellectual infection, poverty), every own family need to be seen as particular in the way those elements have an effect on their ability to defend their person people. Each family's individualized remedy plan will go with the drift logically from the consequences of the complete own family assessment. Therapists want to be cautious not have preconceived thoughts of the dreams of individual households and search for data to verify these ideas. All the to be had statistics should be considered to appearance the way it suits together to provide an explanation for each circle of relatives.

Family Treatment Planning - The following are some commonplace regions that may need to be addressed within the individualized family remedy way:

• Assets and liabilities within the regions of accepting duty, capacity to apprehend issues, and motivation to trade

• Patterns of social interplay, on the aspect of aggressiveness or passivity, the person of contact and involvement with others, the presence or absence of social assist networks and relationships

• Parenting practices (strategies of area, kinds of supervision, understanding of toddler improvement and/or of emotional goals of children)

• Background and records of the dad and mom or caregivers, which includes the facts of abuse and overlook

• Assets and liabilities in the regions of get entry to to simple necessities which incorporates earnings, employment, good enough housing, toddler care, transportation, and wanted offerings and allows

• Behavior/situations related to:

? Domestic violence

? Mental infection

? Physical fitness

? Physical, intellectual, and cognitive disabilities

? Alcohol and drug use

Child and Youth Treatment Planning - Similarly, some of areas of infant and kids functioning furthermore need to be protected into treatment. Depending on age, developmental degree, environment, and family lifestyle, the subsequent need to be tested:

• Physical fitness and motor skills

• Intellectual potential and cognitive functioning

• Academic success

• Emotional and social functioning

• Vulnerability/functionality to talk or guard themselves

• Developmental needs

• Readiness of young adults to transport closer to independence

Multidimensional Treatment - Citing the complexity of treating youngsters and families who have been cited defensive services, Rubin (2012) factors to the want of growing a remedy application that encompasses more than one components tailored to the desires of every circle of relatives. Such additives also can need to encompass interventions for a big sort of troubles together with:

• Disruptive behavior troubles

• Childhood anxiety issues

• Attachment issues

• Trauma-based totally totally dynamics

• Intimate associate violence

• Alcohol and drug abuse

Beyond attention of the wanted components, Rubin (2012) similarly espouses an ecological technique that addresses more than one issues in the course of more than one domains. That is, for intense, lengthy-status and complex clinical problems, the treatment method ought to be as complex because the constellation of supplying problems. This approach is normal with Uri Bronfenbrenner's (1979) principle of social ecology, which holds that more youthful humans are embedded in a couple of systems (figure, family, and social community) and that every one structures have an effect on every notable in reciprocal style. In as a bargain as parental and social structures have an impact on infant and teenagers conduct, children conduct additionally impacts each of those systems.

As an example, think a infant is as an opportunity disruptive at college. The trainer and faculty counselors placed into effect a behavioral intervention, however it is not a hit due to the truth the dad and mom do not comply with thru with domestic-based totally completely outcomes. The dad and mom aren't effective at examine-via because of the fact they're not able to manage their anger, foremost to physical pressure in the direction of the kid. The university specialists forestall the behavioral interventions due to the fact they may be not strolling.

In order to be powerful, behavioral interventions must encompass all worried events – the children, mother and father, college employees, or even network property. Domestic violence without a doubt qualifies as a extreme, extended-status and complicated medical hassle. As such, an individualized multisystemic treatment software need to observe a whole, strengths-based totally absolutely absolutely circle of relatives evaluation.

Part II: Intimate Partner Violence

As is the case with infant abuse, intimate companion violence is a exceptional social problem. In surveys, over 35% of ladies and 28% of fellows say they had been raped and/or physically assaulted and/or stalked by means of using the use of a modern or former accomplice, cohabiting associate, or date at a while in their lifetime (Black et al, 2011). According to the National Intimate Partner and Sexual Violence Survey [NISVS] (Black et al. 2011), "Sexual violence, stalking, and intimate associate violence are principal public health problems inside the United States. Many survivors of these types of violence can revel in physical harm, highbrow fitness effects along facet melancholy, anxiety, low conceitedness, and suicide attempts, and specific health outcomes which includes gastrointestinal troubles, substance abuse, sexually transmitted ailments, and gynecological or pregnancy complications. These consequences can result in hospitalization, disability, or lack of life."

Current findings always suggest that IPV is a pattern, now not an remoted occasion (Fowler and Westen, 2011). "In a nationally consultant sample of 8,000 girls and 8,000 men, elderly 18 and older, the National Violence in opposition to Women Survey mentioned that thirds of ladies bodily assaulted with the aid of a partner were victimized a couple of instances."

One high-quality examine is that there seem to be warning signs and signs that a few sorts of IPV may be at the decline in cutting-edge years. For example, the National Crime Victimization Survey (Truman, 2011) indicated that the fee of intimate partner violence for girls reduced from 4.2

individuals steady with 1,000 in 2009 to three.1 humans consistent with 1,000 in 2010.

Definitions of Terms

Five styles of intimate accomplice violence are described in the NISVS. These include sexual violence, stalking, bodily violence, mental aggression, and control of reproductive/sexual health.

1. Sexual violence consists of rape, being made to penetrate a person else, sexual coercion, unwanted sexual touch, and non-touch unwanted sexual reviews.

2. Physical violence includes loads of behaviors from slapping, pushing or shoving to excessive acts collectively with being beaten, burned, or choked.

3. Stalking victimization includes a pattern of harassing or threatening methods utilized by a wrongdoer that is each unwanted and motives fear or safety troubles inside the victim.

4. Psychological aggression consists of expressive aggression (on the facet of name calling, insulting or humiliating an intimate associate) and coercive

control, which incorporates behaviors which may be imagined to show screen and control or threaten an intimate companion.

five. Control of reproductive or sexual fitness includes the refusal by means of an intimate companion to use a condom. For a female, it's also instances while a associate attempted to get her pregnant while she did no longer want to turn out to be pregnant. For a person, it is also times while a associate tried to get pregnant at the same time as the person did now not want her to come to be pregnant.

Numbers of Victims of IPV

A Word about IPV Statistics

In the way of in search of to collect statistics on what number of human beings are sufferers of IPV, one encounters a dizzying array of disparate numbers. In the give up, it's far based upon on how IPV is defined and what questions are requested. The National Institute of Justice (NIJ), which measures and reports on intimate accomplice violence inside the context of present day crime victimization, states it this manner:

How researchers define terms and pose survey questions topics. Measuring intimate partner violence — frequently referred to as "domestic violence" — can produce surely certainly one of a kind results relying on the gadgets used, the focus of the survey (crime, protection, health) and the severity of injuries. NCVS measures intimate partner violence inside the context of standard crime victimization, and respondents solution with this context in mind. NCVS additionally combines more than one victimizations within a 6-month period if the sufferer isn't always able to remember the facts of each crime, thereby probably undercounting victimizations.

When respondents are asked behaviorally oriented questions, as with the NIJ/Centers for Disease Control and Prevention (CDC)-backed National Violence in the direction of Women Survey (NVAWS), they document higher incidences of intimate accomplice violence.

The trouble receives even more complex. The screening questions used by every survey variety drastically. Moreover, NVAWS is based on random-digit dialing from a database of families that have a cell smartphone and takes precautions to make certain the confidentiality of responses. The NCVS pattern, in evaluation, interviews all individuals of a household who're 12 and older and re-interviews them every 6 months over a 3-year duration, making privateness more hard to maintain.

National Institute of Justice http://www.Nij.Gov/topics/crime/intimate-companion-violence/measuring.Htm - retrieved 2/2/12

The foregoing is included through way of cautioning the reader towards taking any of the information provided in this segment to be definitive representations of the fact of the prevalence of IPV. Nevertheless, some of facts are blanketed herein for the reason of setting up a few experience of the pervasiveness of various elements of IPV. The creator is quite high quality that readers will locate differing – probably even conflicting – records in numerous places some specific vicinity.

Data from the National Intimate Partner and Sexual Violence Survey (NISVS)

Women. More than one-1/three of ladies inside the United States (35.6% or approximately 40 .Four million) have skilled rape, physical violence, and/or stalking by means of manner of an intimate partner sooner or later of their lifetime (Table 5). One in three girls (32.Nine%) has experienced physical violence with the beneficial useful resource of an intimate associate, more than 1 in 10 (10.7%) has been a sufferer of stalking, and nearly 1 in 10 (9.Four%) has been raped thru an intimate partner in her lifetime. Breakdowns via ethnic institution are provided in Table 6.

Men. More than 1 in 4 men within the United States (28.Five%) has professional rape, physical violence, and/or stalking with the aid of an intimate associate in some unspecified time inside the future in their lifetime. Most of the violence said thru approach of men come to be physical violence; best 2.1% stated experiencing stalking through an intimate accomplice (Table 7). Breakdowns with the aid of ethnic group are offered in Table eight.

Victim Profiles: Age

Nearly one-zero.33 of survivors reporting IPV have been 19 – 29 (31.6%). Survivors between 30-39 accounted for close to one 5th (17.Three%) of fashionable records, forty – 40 9 represented nearly 15% (14.Nine%), at the equal time as survivors 50 – fifty nine accounted for six.Four%. Survivors who did not reveal their age represented 19.Nine%. Survivors older than 60 only accounted for two.Eight% of overall survivors (Table nine).

Victim Profiles: Race/Ethnicity

White sufferers accounted for nearly a 3rd (29.Five%) of normal survivors and Latina/o diagnosed survivors accounted for 1 / 4 (25.1%) of common survivors. Black/African American survivors made up 10.Three% of survivors and multi-racial survivors accounted for 4.7% of great survivors.

Asian/Pacific Islander survivors made up 4.2% of survivors and self-identified survivors accounted for three.Four% of the entire. Arab/Middle-Eastern (0.Eight%), Indigenous/ First People (zero.Eight%), and South Asian (0.1%) survivors comprised much less than 5% of the complete facts (Table 10).

IPV inside Lesbian, Gay, Bisexual, Transgender, Queer, and HIV-Affected (LGBTQH) Communities

There is exceptional constrained studies at the question of intimate accomplice violence inside lesbian, homosexual, bisexual, transgender, queer, and HIV-affected (LGBTQH) groups. Thanks to a modern-day document by means of manner of the National Coalition of Anti-Violence Programs (NCAVP, 2010), there within the period in-between are a few initial information to be had. NCAVP produces the every year LGBTQH Intimate Partner Violence Report to provide special data on intimate partner violence interior LGBTQH companies, highlight essential issues, and present hints to insurance makers and network contributors.

There are first-rate limitations on conclusions that may be crafted from the statistics on this report. First, thinking about they were gathered from people who self-cautioned and from different public resources, those numbers do no longer represent all incidents of intimate companion violence in opposition to LGBTQH humans inside the United States. Therefore, even as the information contained in this file affords an in depth photo of the individual survivors who noted to NCAVP member applications, it can't and ought to not be extrapolated to symbolize the overall LGBTQH population inside the United States. Second, for the reason that there are not any dependable statistics at the numbers of humans in each LGBTQH class inside the fashionable population, it isn't always viable to make any much less high priced comparisons the various ones agencies and the general populace. Nevertheless, the facts accrued do provide a few provisional insights into IPV in LGBTQH groups.

In a literature evaluation, Carvalho et al. (2011) stated an array of information that serves to demonstrate the sizable levels and conflicting findings which have been available till very currently:

Recent evaluations record occurrence estimates starting from 17% to fifty two% (Ristock 2005), and among 25% and 50% (Murray and Mobley 2009) in gay and lesbian relationships. Some research suggest that same-intercourse IPV takes location at a fee that is similar or decrease to charges of heterosexual partner violence (e.G., Brand and Kidd 1986; Gardner 1989; Tjaden and

Thoennes 2000a), whilst others determined a better incidence of IPV in equal-intercourse relationships (Balsam et al. 2005; Tjaden and Thoennes 2000b; Turell 2000).

It appears easy that now not something might be very clear at this point.

Definitions (APA, 2009, p. 28)

Gender Identity - refers to a person's easy revel in of being male, female, or of indeterminate intercourse.

Sexual Orientation - refers back to the tendency to be sexually inquisitive about ladies and men of the same sex, the opportunity intercourse, each sexes, or neither intercourse.

Transgender or Gender Variant - refers back to the behavior, look, or identity of ladies and men who flow into, transcend, or do not agree to culturally described norms for parents in their biological sex.

Genderqueer - generally used as a capture-all or umbrella term for folks who pick out themselves as some aspect other than person, along with each guy and lady (intersex) or neither guy nor female.

Victim Profiles: Gender Identity

Female sufferers account for almost half of (45.7%) of IPV instances stated to NCAVP in 2010, with male survivors accounting for greater than a 3rd (36.Eight%). Transgender survivors comprised four.2% (1.2% transgender guys and 3.Zero% transgender girls) of fashionable survivors. Eleven% of survivors did not divulge their gender identification. Genderqueer (0.1%), intersex (0.Five%), and self-diagnosed (1.7%) human beings make up tons much less than 5% of enormous survivors.

Victim Profiles: Sexual Orientation

Victims were the most in all likelihood to understand as either Gay (31.Five%) or Lesbian (28.Three%). Bisexual survivors accounted for nine.Three% of widespread survivors. Heterosexual survivors accounted for eight.Zero% of desired survivors on the equal time as 18.Four% of survivors did now not disclose their sexual orientation. Questioning (1.1%), Queer (1.Eight%), and Self-identified (1.2%) survivors comprised less than 5% of the complete information (Figure four).

A word on institutionalized bias. The NCVAP (2010) survey determined out that a excessive range (40 four.6%) of LGBTQH survivors have been have become away from intimate companion violence shelters. This stunning statistic highlights the impact of institutionalized discrimination on LGBTQH groups and has a proper away impact on LGBTQH survivors' get admission to to help and services. According to the file, "LGBTQH survivors aren't receiving the vital manual they need once they do are seeking out help. Institutional homophobic, biphobic, and transphobic bias and discrimination deter many LGBTQH survivors from engaging in out for beneficial resource to begin with" (NCAVP, 2010).

Perpetrators of Intimate Partner Violence

Perpetrator Profiles: Relationship to Victim

Most patients of rape understand their perpetrators. According to the NISVS (Black et al. 2011):

• More than 1/2 (fifty one.1%) of female patients of rape noted that at the least one perpe¬trator changed into a modern-day or former intimate companion

• Four out of 10 (40.Eight%) of female sufferers stated being raped by means of an acquaintance.

• About 1 in 7 girl patients (thirteen.Eight%) suggested being raped with the resource of the usage of a stranger.

• Approximately 1 in 8 (12.Five%) female patients pronounced being raped by manner of a member of the family

• 2.Five% said being raped with the aid of someone in a function of authority.

Perpetrator Profiles: Psychiatric Correlates

As a part of a larger National Institute of Mental Health (NIMH)–funded mission, an modern check (Fowler and Westen 2011) accomplished a modern-day method to derive subtypes of male perpetrators of intimate companion violence. A national pattern of randomly decided on psychologists and psychiatrists describe 188 grownup male sufferers, of whom fifty nine had a statistics of accomplice violence. Results indicated an association among violence and each melancholy and substance abuse. In the sample of partner-violence perpetrators, 28.Eight% have been identified with essential melancholy, and 39.Zero% with substance use issues. With admire to Axis II diagnoses, 66.Zero% met standards for antisocial PD (APD), 40 four.1% for paranoid PD, 27.1% for borderline PD (BPD), sixteen.Nine% for avoidant PD, and 8.Five% for based PD (Table 12)

The authors have been able to deliver collectively a composite portrait of the common companion-violent man inside the sample. The portrait became "marked through using anger, impulsivity, and alienation. Interpersonally, the not unusual accomplice-violent guy have become characterized as having few near relationships, being touchy to complaint and having a bent to maintain grudges, involved in energy struggles, and essential and controlling. They tended to be emotionally dysregulated, impulsive, lacking in belief, and prone to feeling misunderstood, mistreated, or victimized (Fowler and Westen, 2011). This constellation of tendencies is probably taken thru the usage of clinicians as a red flag in preserving vigilance in competition to IPV in medical exercise.